The
EASY EATING DIET

Make Healthy Eating Easy
and Lose the Weight
and Food Guilt Forever!

SEAN BARKER, CPT, PN2

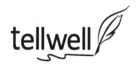

Tellwell Talent
www.tellwell.ca

ISBN
978-1-77370-981-9 (Hardcover)
978-1-77370-982-6 (Paperback)
978-1-77370-980-2 (eBook)

To Dad, for letting me find my passion and purpose.

To Mom, for always providing me a soft place to fall.

To my wife Kathy, for your patience, love and support.

To Matea and Caden, for giving me a bigger reason why.

*To all my family and friends who have
supported me along the way.*

DISCLAIMER

You must get your physicians approval before beginning this eating or exercise program. These recommendations are not medical guidelines but are for educational purposes only. You must consult your physician prior to starting this program or if you have any medical condition or injury that contraindicates diet changes or physical activity. This program is designed for healthy individuals 18 years and older only.

The information in this book is meant to supplement, not replace, proper nutrition and exercise programming. All forms of exercise pose some inherent risks. The editors and publishers advise readers to take full responsibility for their safety and know their limits. Before practicing the exercises in this book, do not take risks beyond your level of experience, aptitude, training and fitness. The exercises and dietary programs in this book are not intended as a substitute for any exercise routine or treatment or dietary regimen that may have been prescribed by your physician.

See your physician before starting any exercise or nutrition program. If you are taking any medications, you must talk to your physician before starting any exercise or eating program. If you experience any lightheadedness, dizziness, or shortness of breath while exercising, stop the movement and consult a physician. You must have a complete physical examination if you are sedentary, if you have high cholesterol, high blood pressure, or diabetes, if you are overweight, or if you are over 30 years old. Please discuss all nutritional changes with your physician or a registered dietician.

CONTENTS

ABOUT THE AUTHOR

Sean Barker is a husband, father of two, foodie and fitness coach. Some career highlights include:

- President of Valley Fit Body Bootcamp Inc.
- Contributing writer for many mainstream fitness publications such as Men's Health and Inside Fitness magazine.

Sean rises up at 4 am every morning with energy and enthusiasm and has a burning desire for self-development, being a health hacker and over the last 23 years, has traveled the world to learn from the best in the fitness industry.

Through this time Sean has been successful coaching clients through body transformations online with his various information products like Dad Fitness, 6 Week Fat Loss Blueprint, his own cookbook, Fit Body Food and and now this book, the Easy Eating Diet.

Offline he owns and operates KV Fit Body Bootcamp in New Brunswick Canada where along with his team, coaches busy parents and professionals to be their best Fit Body.

Sean was nominated by his industry peers for Personal Trainer of the Year in 2015 and 2018 at Fitness Business Summit in California. He was a keynote speaker at the same event the previous year. He has also spoken twice on stage at the Fit Body Bootcamp

Franchise World Conference and for many other companies and organizations.

In 2014 he was voted 3rd place in North America for the Men's Health Next Top Trainer contest and selected by Men's Health as one of their MVP contributing fitness writers.

He is also a current contributing writer to Canada's leading fitness magazine, Inside Fitness.

In 2001 Sean was the first from his hometown of Wabush, Labrador, Canada to compete provincially in bodybuilding and also received runner-up in the world-wide AST Sports Science Body Transformation Contest, appearing in their High Performance Muscle Magazine and receiving a sports supplement endorsement contract.

Sean loves motivating in person but also through the written word and his email newsletters have been called by his clients "the best thing I read to start my day along with my morning coffee".

He has also been awarded Top 10 business owner and received the golden franchise success award by Fit Body Bootcamp franchise headquarters.

Sean believes "every day is a chance to get better", for himself as a coach, as well as his clients. He continues to be driven to succeed in spreading his passion for achieving health and happiness.

PREFACE

THE PERFECT DIET

Calories in versus calories out. Eat less, move more. The perfect pill, potion or percentage. Eat real foods. Eat clean foods. High protein. Low carbohydrate. High fat ... The ideas and the advice go on and on.

Easy to say, but not so easy to do, right? Confusing? Yes!

And this is just a fraction of the type of advice you get when you ask someone about the D word—the word DIET.

If I had any hair left on my head I would pull it out and scream. Do you feel the same way about finding the perfect diet?

When did eating and controlling our weight and health get so confusing? And more importantly, when will the confusion stop?

Well, hopefully it stops right now, the minute you begin reading this book. I want you to know you've made a smart decision in purchasing this book and that *Easy Eating* will be the best companion and guide to a new you that you have ever had. That's because *Easy Eating* is not a a diet book at all, at least not as far as the word diet is commonly defined in the Oxford English dictionary:

DIET:

> "to restrict oneself to small amounts or special kinds of food in order to lose weight."
>
> "a special course of food to which one restricts oneself, either to lose weight or for medical reasons."

For most people, 'dieting' ends with failure and discouragement. Despite an initial high from short-term weight-loss results, the average calorie-restricted dieter ends up hating their life after a few weeks or months and eventually quits 'dieting' when the lure of their favorite foods and the frustration of preparing complicated recipes becomes too much to bear.

Ultimately the dieter returns to eating the way they did in the past—and they return to the same body weight as well, sometimes to a higher weight than before.

But worse for a person than gaining back the weight are the residual feelings of frustration and failure left lingering after each diet attempt, feelings that push the dieter farther and farther away from his or her best body, discouraging them from finding a real, permanent solution.

Yet there is another definition of 'diet' that many don't think of when they hear that word— and that's the definition used in this book.

When I refer to 'diet' in this book I mean:

DIET:

> "The kinds of food that a person, animal, or community habitually eats."

That's it. 'Diet' is just a word for the foods we all eat. So I think we can all relax a little.

This book doesn't advocate for or promote certain foods. There are no 'good' or 'bad' foods; no diet dogma or extreme food restrictions. Every food (unless you have a serious food allergy) in the *Easy Eating Diet* is fair game to eat and all you have to do is follow some simple science strategies, practical principles and healthy hacks.

In today's nutrition realm there is, unfortunately, very little reliable research happening that addresses what most of us care about when we think of diets: getting leaner and lighter. Most of the money spent on nutritional research is spent on studying disease prevention and analyzing health markers. Which is great! But it's not helpful for those of us who are more interested in looking good on the beach.

That's why, in this book, we are going to get back to proven and practical strategies for healthy weight loss and fat loss (not always the same thing, you will discover).

We will wipe the plate clean, so to speak, and clear the confusion on carbohydrates; examine the shocking truth about the numbers on the scale; get the goods on gluten; and, eliminate the highs and lows that diets cause when they lead you down a dead-end street, leaving you with nothing but a light wallet and heavy heart.

You'll learn proven how-to hacks for building healthy habits for life as well as new tips and tricks about how to make eating easier— all without the white-knuckle willpower, extreme food restriction and constant decision fatigue that are part of diets that cause you to worry about what to eat every single day.

You will discover and use the latest neuroscience research about lifestyle and behavioral change to finally make healthy habits stick. Because it's not just what you know ... it's are you *doing* what you know?

Further, you'll uncover the mistakes we all make with our mindset and motivation and you'll learn how to implement your new skills and knowledge in the context of real life as a busy parent or professional.

Plus, you will get our meals in minutes recipes and meal planning guides to make eating easy and enjoyable without spending hours in the kitchen.

Finally, a way to start feeling great, to lose unwanted weight and to gain freedom from food, forever!

But I don't want you to just read this book. I want you to practice it.

Keep this book where you can always see it, like on your kitchen counter, your coffee table or your desk at work. Not only is it a good reminder to keep your eating easy and to stay on track with your goals, but you can use it for reference and return to when the next diet fad gets pushed your way, because it will.

I hope this book will be a guiding light to clarity and confidence moving forward and that it helps you to finally achieve the health and happiness you deserve, with the food you eat and the life you live.

INTRODUCTION

THE BIG FAT TRUTH

It was the early 90s and I remember my father coming home from his company's annual medical checkup, disturbed to learn that his cholesterol was high.

What didn't add up was that my father then only in his 40s, was actually very fit and worked out regularly. He was a fixture in our local gym and swimming pool and he liked to go for runs outside in our small, isolated hometown of Wabush, Labrador, in Northern Canada during the short and much-savored summer months.

At 170 pounds and five feet, seven inches tall my father certainly wasn't overweight or unfit but after his checkup, left with news of his high cholesterol (which at that time was popping up all over the news as being the big health marker to keep in check) he was worried. After all, high cholesterol was being touted as the main contributor to heart disease and the way to prevent it was to follow a low-fat diet.

So, in an honest attempt to follow his doctor's advice and my mother's obvious concern, it wasn't long before all the food in our house was magically replaced with low-fat forms of their evil, fattening cousins that previously stocked the cupboard.

And as the low-fat food trend popularity soared, food marketers didn't stop at offering just low-fat items; they kept topping themselves by selling multiple versions of the same products, with 40 percent less fat, 60 percent less fat ... even products that were supposed to be primarily fat by nature, like mayonnaise, were now available—with 0 percent fat!

High-fat eggs, bacon and butter were out; low-fat cereal, toast and margarine were in. Of course all of this was to be washed down with a tall glass of sugary orange juice, which Saturday morning TV constantly reminded us was, 'part of a complete healthy breakfast!'

Why did no one ever stop to ask, 'what are they replacing all the natural fats in these foods with? Is it really any better? Could it even be worse?'

As a teenager I developed a passion for health and fitness, thanks to working out with my Dad. But after picking up my first muscle magazine and seeing that food was no longer just food but a complicated calculation of calories, protein, carbohydrates and fats I was reluctantly introduced to this not-so wonderful world of 'meal math' that turned the ease of eating good, normal food into something difficult and hard to understand.

Math was always my most despised subject in school, but it seemed it was now needed to calculate nutritional food facts, fat grams and count calories on the back of food labels.

I remember my grandmother (who lived to be 93 and was never overweight), chuckling at me once when she saw me reading the nutrition facts on the back of a box of chicken breasts as she asked, "what are you reading? it's just food!"

I think we can learn something from her.

With my father's dedication to this new low-fat diet he quickly lost about 10 pounds off his already-fit frame, which made him actually look sick, not healthier, as well as almost ten years older. He was lethargic at work and had little energy left for his workouts.

Friends and family began to notice too and started to ask if he was sick and wondering was he even battling a disease.

Then the moment of truth came when he went back to the doctor a few months later to get his cholesterol re-checked. Everyone was confident that by making the recommended changes in his diet that had been prescribed by the doctor (bearing in mind that his diet wasn't really bad to begin with) that he would be in the normal cholesterol range and as healthy on the inside as he was known for being on the outside.

Unfortunately that wasn't the case; after all that sacrifice and low-fat eating, his cholesterol numbers didn't go down one bit. I remember seeing the frustration on his then-frail face when he came home from this follow-up check-up. He had listened to the doctors and media about the importance of lowering cholesterol to prevent heart disease and done what they told him to do—giving up food he loved to eat for low-fat food with no success. The only thing the medical establishment had left to offer him now was cholesterol-lowering drugs.

This could have been disheartening, and my father might have lost faith in food companies and dieting after that, but instead he got back to eating his normal healthy diet, exercising consistently and eventually he returned to his normal, healthy weight. He focused on what he knew he could control and began doing research about cholesterol. What he found out was that very little of a person's diet affects blood serum cholesterol in the body and—even more shocking—most medical doctors only receive an average of 20 hours of nutrition education during their many years of study. And so it seemed possible that he had been given wrong information about the relationship between diet and heart health.

This revelation is not his alone; with billions of dollars pumping the food marketing machine, we are left with our hands out of the cookie jar and up in the air with paralysis by analysis, not knowing what to do and what to believe anymore. We have seen the trends go from from high-carbohydrate to low-fat, to low-carbohydrate, to high-protein and now high-fat (such as the keto diet) in the most recent years.

But where has this diet roller coaster gotten us over the last hundred years? Nowhere! There is an obesity epidemic, particularly in North America, and people are fatter, heavier and sicker as a society than ever before, despite all the food science and fitness technology available to us.

Should we really be getting our nutritional guidance from doctors, news anchors and social media clickbait? Cultures around the world have survived and eaten intuitively for millions of years without the knowledge and science we have today and have thrived. Yet we seem confused. Is it because we are constantly hammered with contradictory and ever-changing guidelines along with miracle cures for our muffin tops that include popping pills, potions and proper percentages?

We now spend more time in cubicles than caves and we are not out hunting and growing our food. Our society and food landscape has drastically changed in the last hundred years, and our senses are assaulted with colorful packaging and better tastes, our bellies easily filled with immediately accessible, processed foods—but our basic biological need for nourishment has changed very little from the needs of our ancestors before us.

It's time we take back control of our diet, our health, and our happiness by simplifying something that has been made far too complicated and cumbersome for too many years. Let's make eating easy again, but at the same time ensuring that we give our body what it needs while still giving our emotional self the enjoyment of eating what we want. Yes, food is fuel, but it is okay to eat for pure pleasure at times.

Unlike other diets that demonize certain food groups and serve them up with a side of diet dogma, the *Easy Eating Diet* is like a 'choose your own adventure' book. It is a guide that can keep you in control of your journey towards better health by allowing you the flexibility you need to enjoy eating for health and weight loss along with the enjoyment of eating for pleasure—but without the heavy food guilt (which is sometimes worse than the food itself!) Plus you will be provided with simple strategies you can put to use today to develop rock-solid, healthy habits for life.

You and I will be on this journey together; you will always be the leader. Choosing and knowing where you want to go. The *Easy Eating Diet* will be the roadmap to help guide you and get you there, mentally and physically. The book has strategies to get you back on track if you ever feel lost and to make sure you actually enjoy the journey along the way. Crazy concept, right?

I am confident the *Easy Eating Diet* is the last diet book you will ever need, because it's not really a diet book at all. Further, it's also a lot more than merely a book on eating for health, happiness and weight loss; the purpose of this book is to empower you with mental and physical success strategies, not just about eating and exercise, but on being your best self wherever you currently are—and wherever you want to go.

Unlike so many other diet plans that leave you with no power to choose how to eat and don't teach life-long skills that fit your lifestyle, *The Easy Eating Diet* will give you back the three's C's: Choice, Confidence and Control. Now that sounds like a plan!

> "Sometimes the food guilt is worse than the food itself."
>
> —Sean Barker

CHAPTER 1:
SIMPLE SCIENCE

THE POWER OF PROTEIN AND PIZZA

The macronutrient protein is popular and has been written about in many diet books over the years, but there is one thing to remember and realize about protein: it is an essential building block of life. So yeah, it's critical you get enough protein in your diet.

The word protein comes from the Greek word *proteos*, meaning the 'first one,' or the 'most important one.' Plus, the Ancient Greeks seem to have invented pizza, so they must have known a thing or two about food.

Proteins are crucial to healthy human biological processes.

The human body stores vital information inside some proteins; still others are involved in muscle contraction and critical immune responses. Even when we learn something, it happens through changes in protein structures within the neurons of our brains. We grow, we change and live our entire lives due to processes in our body that are reliant on proteins. Pretty important stuff, that protein.

Here is some simple science: all animal and plant proteins on earth are constructed from only 20 different amino acids. Think of amino acids as train cars that make up an entire train called a protein. Nine of these 20 amino acids are known as 'essential amino acids. Essential amino acids cannot be made by the body. As a result, they must come from food.

These nine essential amino acids obtained through food are vital because some key metabolic processes to create energy and provide the basic building blocks needed for growth and repair. need protein enzymes in order to occur. You must consume protein so you can make more protein enzymes.

In terms of helping to whittle down your waistline, protein starts its magic the moment it leaves your fork. Of the three macro-nutrients in our food—protein, carbohydrates and fats—protein is the most 'thermogenic,' meaning our bodies burn up more calories just to digest and assimilate protein.

Protein is also more satiating and smaller portions fill a person up more than carbohydrates or fat do. For example, most of us couldn't sit down and eat three or four steaks at a sitting, even if they *were* only the size of our palm (the recommended serving), because steaks are comprised of protein and some fat, which fills us up. But we *could* sit down and eat three or four slices of bread the size of our palm (mostly carbohydrates) if we were really hungry.

When you eat natural protein based foods, you don't have to stress so much about perfect portions because it's very hard to overeat. Mother nature knew what she was doing when she created plants and animals, we just stopped listening to her, like we do with our own mothers. Sorry Mom! Plus staying full and satisfied and avoiding getting 'hangry' is the key to any sustain-able way of eating.

In a study published in the research journal Nutrition Metabolism, dieters who increased their protein intake to 30 percent of their diet ate nearly 450 fewer calories a day and lost about 11 pounds over a 12-week study period without employing any other dietary measures.

Protein is also essential for making sure you lose fat, not muscle (your metabolic engine). Your body uses the amino acids in protein to build lean muscle, which not only makes you stronger and leaner but also burns calories even when you're not active—unlike fat. Ultimately, this keeps your metabolism humming along at high speed so you can burn off the occasional cookie, no problem.

For anyone who is exercising, and especially incorporating resistance training into their exercise routine, protein is crucial to the metabolic processes of muscle repair and recovery. That muscle soreness you feel from overdoing it a little in the gym won't just magically go away. It's the power of protein plus time that will help you recover.

A Johns Hopkins University study found that a diet in which roughly 25 percent of the calories came from lean protein sources helped reduce blood pressure, LDL (low-density lipoprotein or "bad") cholesterol levels and triglycerides better than a traditional higher-carbohydrate diet. Other research has found that diets rich in protein can help prevent obesity, osteoporosis, and diabetes.

I think you get the point. Protein is important, even on pizza.

FIVE HEALTHY HACKS TO EAT MORE PROTEIN

1. **Simple Supplement.** Supplementing your diet with a high-quality protein powder such as a whey or plant-based one is an easy way to consume 20 to 30 grams of protein per scoop. Look for a brand with minimal additional ingredients preferably one that is naturally sweetened with stevia. Blend it in a smoothie or mix it into food. Or opt for

an easy grab-and-go high-quality protein bar containing whey or plant protein as its main protein source. Read the labels as many supposedly healthy protein bars are chocked full of cheap, processed soy protein and additional sugar.

2. **Easy Eggs.** One whole egg contains six grams of protein. Half the protein is in the yolk along with many other nutrients so I recommend consuming some yolks. But to boost the protein content in your meal to 20-30 grams with minimal calories and with less egg-cracking fuss, you can add in some liquid egg whites to your scramble or omelet. Egg whites are pure, ready- to-pour protein.

3. **Super Seeds.** As convenient snacks or sprinkled into your food, pumpkin seeds, de-shelled soft hemp seeds (known as hemp hearts) or chia seeds are all high in plant protein (around 10 to 15 grams of protein per serving) that comes paired with some healthy omega-3 fats and fiber to give your meals and daily diet a little more protein power.

4. **Do Dairy.** If you have no digestive issues consuming dairy products like milk, cheese and Greek yogurt, then dairy is a tasty and easy way to add some slow-digesting and filling protein to your diet.

5. **Sensible Starch.** Again, if you have no digestive issues consuming beans and legumes, these, along with other ancient grains like quinoa, are fairly high in plant protein (15 to 20 grams of protein per serving). Just watch the portions if you are watching your weight ,as they are higher in carbohydrates compared to animal-based proteins, which are composed only of protein and fat.

CHAPTER 2:
PERFECT PLANTS

From a young age most of us are made aware of the health benefits of eating fruits and vegetables. We learn it from our parents at the dinner table when we are made to wrestle the Jolly Green Giant of greens left on our plate and we learn it in school coloring the rainbow of fruit flavors.

It's well-known that fruits and vegetables have many health benefits. A wide range of research supports and indicates that a diet high in fruits and vegetables is beneficial to heart health, can lower diabetes and cancer risk and may improve brain function.

A diet rich in fruits and vegetables can also lower blood pressure, reduce risk of stroke, prevent some types of cancer, lower risk of eye and digestive problems and have a positive effect upon blood sugar, which can help keep appetites in check.

Fruits and vegetables are an important part of a healthy diet and they also provide the powerful benefit of variety and choice. However, no single fruit or vegetable provides all the nutrients you need to be healthy.

Green vegetables, with their high nutrient content but extremely low calorie and carbohydrate count, can almost be considered 'negative calories,' as your body burns up many of the calories when digesting them. Eat green, get lean.

Try dark leafy greens, then shake things up with brightly colored red, yellow and orange vegetables and fruits. Enjoy cooked tomatoes. Choose color when you can. Eat a variety of types and colors in order to give your body the mix of nutrients it needs. Eat what you enjoy!

DEFENSE AGAINST DISEASE

Cardiovascular disease

There is compelling evidence that a diet rich in fruits and vegetables can lower the risk of heart disease and stroke. The largest and longest study to date, done as part of the Harvard-based Nurses' Health Study in 1976 and the Health Professionals Follow-up Study in 1986 at the Harvard Public School of Health, looked at the health and dietary habits of almost 110,000 men and women over a span of 14 years.

The higher the average daily intake of fruits and vegetables, the lower the chances of developing cardiovascular disease study subjects had. Those who averaged eight or more servings a day were 30 percent less likely to have had a heart attack or stroke during the study period than those in the lowest category of fruit and vegetable intake (less than 1.5 servings a day).

Although all fruits and vegetables likely contribute to this benefit, green leafy vegetables such as lettuce, spinach, Swiss chard and mustard greens; cruciferous vegetables such as broccoli, cauliflower, cabbage, Brussels sprouts, bok choy, and kale; and citrus fruits such as oranges, lemons, limes, and grapefruit (and their juices) make important contributions.

When researchers combined findings from the Harvard studies with several other long-term studies in the U.S. and Europe, and looked at coronary heart disease and stroke separately, they found a similar protective effect: individuals who ate more than five servings of fruits and vegetables per day had roughly a 20 percent lower risk of coronary heart disease and stroke, compared with individuals who ate less than three servings per day.

Blood pressure

The Dietary Approaches to Stop Hypertension (DASH) study done by the National Institute of Health (NIH) in 1992 worked with five of the most well-respected medical research centers in different cities across the U.S. and conducted the largest and most detailed research study to date. They examined the effect on blood pressure of a diet rich in fruits, vegetables and low-fat dairy products that restricted the amount of saturated and total fat. The researchers found that people with high blood pressure who followed this diet reduced their systolic blood pressure (the upper number of a blood pressure reading) by about 11 mm Hg (mmHg being millimeters of mercury) and their diastolic blood pressure (the lower number) by almost 6 mm Hg—as much as medications can achieve.

Cancer

Numerous early studies reveal what appears to be a strong link between eating fruits and vegetables and protection against cancer. Unlike case-control studies, (which rely on observations of past information), cohort studies, which follow large groups of initially healthy individuals for years, generally provide more reliable information than case-control studies because they don't rely on information from the past. And, in general, data from cohort studies have not consistently shown that a diet rich in fruits and vegetables prevents cancer.

A 2008 report by the World Cancer Research Fund and the American Institute for Cancer Research suggests that non-starchy vegetables—such as lettuce and other leafy greens, broccoli, bok choy, cabbage, as well as garlic, onions, and fruits "probably" protect against several types of cancers.

A line of research stemming from a finding from the Health Professionals Follow-up Study suggests that tomatoes may help protect men against prostate cancer, especially aggressive forms of it. One of the pigments that give tomatoes their red hue—lycopene—could be involved in this protective effect. Although several studies other than the Health Professionals study have also demonstrated a link between tomatoes or lycopene and prostate cancer, others have not or have found only a weak connection.

Taken as a whole, however, these studies suggest that increased consumption of tomato-based products (especially cooked tomato products) and other lycopene-containing foods may reduce the occurrence of prostate cancer. Lycopene is one of several carotenoids (compounds that the body can turn into vitamin A) found in brightly colored fruits and vegetables, and research suggests that foods containing carotenoids may protect against lung, mouth, and throat cancer. But more research is needed before we know the exact relationship between fruits and vegetables, carotenoids, and cancer.

Diabetes

Some research looks specifically at whether individual fruits are associated with risk of type 2 diabetes. While there isn't an abundance of research into this area yet, preliminary results are compelling.

Initiated in 1976 and expanded in 1989 at Harvard School of Public Health and Brigham Women's Hospital in Boston, Massachusetts., a study of over 66,000 women in the Nurses' Health Study, 85,104 women from the Nurses' Health Study II, and 36,173 men from the Health Professionals Follow-up Study who were free of major chronic diseases, findings suggested that greater consumption of whole fruits – especially blueberries, grapes, and apples – is associated with a lower risk of type 2 diabetes.

Another important finding, but not surprising, (as fiber found in whole fruit helps mitigate blood sugar spikes) is that greater consumption of fruit juice is associated with a higher risk of type 2 diabetes.

Additionally, a 2008 report in Diabetes Care looked at over 70,000 female nurses aged 38-63 years who were free of cardiovascular disease, cancer, and diabetes, research showed that consumption of green leafy vegetables and fruit was associated with a lower risk of diabetes.

A Kuopio Ischaemic Heart Disease Risk Factor Study in 1984-1989 of over 2,300 Finnish men showed that fruit and vegetables, especially berries, may reduce the risk of Type 2 diabetes.

Gut Health

Fruits and vegetables contain indigestible fiber, which absorbs water and expands as it passes through the digestive system. This can calm symptoms of an irritable bowel and, by triggering regular bowel movements, can relieve or prevent constipation.

Vision

Eating fruits and vegetables can also keep your eyes healthy and may help prevent two common aging-related eye diseases—cataracts and macular degeneration—which afflict millions of Americans over age 65. Two carotenoids found in fruits and vegetables, Lutein and zeaxanthin, in particular, seem protective against cataracts.

So instead of fighting over all the other diets out there and trying to determine which one is best, I think we should focus on the main thing they have in common: eating plants is just good for us.

FIVE HEALTHY HACKS TO EAT MORE PLANTS

1. **Front and Centre**. Keep fruits and vegetables where you can see them. For example, display apples and bananas on the counter and fresh veggies on the main shelves in your fridge instead of keeping them tucked away in the bottom black hole of the vegetable crisper, never to be seen again until rotten and ready to toss. Shop and chop some of your whole veggies as soon as you bring them home from the supermarket so they are ready to use when you are rushed. Keep them visible and easily accessible and you'll be more likely to use vegetables for easy eating meal prep or a quick grab-and-go snack instead of finding your hand in the bottom of a bag or box of chips or crackers.

2. **Mix it Up.** Explore the produce aisle of your local supermarket or farmer's market and choose something new each week, or at least each month. Make dinner a fun, friends-and-family affair or join a supper club. Cooking with other people will encourage you to find a recipe using new food items as the main star of whatever dish you cook. Variety is the key to a healthy diet, and yes, the spice of life.

3. **Carbohydrates are Cool.** Yes, you can still eat the starchy higher carbohydrate vegetables and tubers that grow in the ground, such as potatoes, onions and carrots. They are packed with nutrients. Different variations of squash are also great and are naturally lower in carbohydrates than most starchy vegetables. Just pair it on your plate with

a palm size portion of protein. Again, it's hard to overeat earth-grown food.

4. **Make it a Meal.** Try cooking new recipes that use vegetables as fillers instead of as a stand-alone side dish. For example, salads, stir-fries, casseroles and even omelets are easy eating ways for sneaking produce onto your plate. Try throwing a handful of baby spinach or kale into some of your everyday meals. Baby greens almost wilt away during cooking due to their high moisture content and you will barely notice they are there. Or try tossing spinach or kale into a blended berry protein smoothie. Once it's pulverized you won't even taste it.

5. **One Pan Plan.** Line a baking pan with parchment paper and bake your favorite vegetables. Prepare them by washing, chopping and peeling, then drizzle them with olive oil, sprinkle with salt, pepper and garlic powder, toss to coat and roast in the oven for 30 to 40 minutes at 400 degrees Fahrenheit or until golden brown. Asparagus, Brussels sprouts, broccoli, cauliflower, potatoes, bell peppers, onions and tomatoes all taste great this way. You can even get frozen, pre-cut vegetables for easier cooking and convenience. It's a fuss-free way to cook a big batch of veggies and have them ready as side dishes. While you're at it, use the other rack and roast some meat at the same time.

> "Eat food. Not too much. Mostly plants."
>
> —Michael Pollan, Author of Food Rules

CHAPTER 3:
CLEAR THE CARBOHYDRATE CONFUSION

So where are the carbohydrates with this *Easy Eating Diet*? Actually there are plenty of nutrient-rich and filling carbohydrates in fruits and vegetables, just not as much per serving as there are in starchier foods.

If you are wondering where the common comfort carbohydrates like breads, pastas, cereals, and grains come into play, as they sound like the outsider in this *Easy Eating Diet*, here is where they stand.

Technically, carbohydrates are not an essential macronutrient for our body like protein or fats. Human's thrived for millions of years with little grain available to them before agriculture was invented. Yet they did harvest wild grains and other wild starches, such as various tubers. So *the Easy Eating Diet* has a place in it for some starchy carbohydrates.

However, unlike the popular and restrictive no-carbohydrate Keto diet, low-carbohydrate and Paleo diet trends that shun most carbohydrates, *The Easy Eating Diet* falls somewhere in the middle, using those diets only as a template to customize carbohydrate limits to food preference and goals. *The Easy Eating Diet* suggests you be 'Smart about Starch' depending on two factors:

1. **Your Activity**

2. **Your Health**

It's not appropriate to demonize any food group in order to lose weight and be healthy despite what other diets may recommend. I don't like to call carbohydrates good carbohydrates or bad carbohydrates, or any food 'good' or 'bad' as food has no moral value (only the moral values we put on them). Just look at what is the best choice to achieve your goals at any given time.

1. **Your Activity Level.** If you are active and lean already, you can eat more carbohydrates without storing it as excess body fat because you are using and burning up more carbohydrates due to higher activity levels and more active muscle tissue.

2. **Your Health.** Do you have digestion or food sensitivity issues? Do you have health issues like cardiovascular disease or diabetes? Do you have specific body composition goals like general weight loss, or more advanced fat loss so you can see your abs staring back at you in the mirror?

The truth about starches and foods high in carbohydrates is that they are just very high in energy, energy that we, as a less active society with less lean bodies than our ancestors, are not burning due to sluggish resting metabolic rates created by sitting on our rumps most of the day staring at computers.

For most people, eating high-carbohydrate food is like filling up a car with gas when the needle is still on full. Ultimately it will overspill. When we eat more than we burn, we gain weight. And this goes for all food and all macronutrients; protein, carbohydrates and fats all contain calories, and for weight loss, calories matter most.

However, regarding carbohydrates, starchy higher-carbohydrate food like bread, pasta and grain are also very easy to overeat. Especially when they come in the form of popular processed snack foods full of the too-good trifecta of salt, sugar and starch. Add lots of fat to that equation and you wind up with an addictive taste that is a bonanza for food marketing companies. These types of food make you want to eat more and buy more. It's hard to eat one potato chip, one French fry or even one small slice of pizza, right?

From a health standpoint, starchy carbohydrate foods—the most common form of processed convenience foods—also contain far fewer micronutrients or vitamins and minerals per serving than their more natural plant-based cousins. Besides spiking our blood sugar, due to the fast digestion of the simple sugars found in more processed starchy carbohydrates, which contributes to obesity, diabetes and insulin resistance, carbohydrate-dense processed foods are very easy to overeat due to their form and convenience, causing many of us to chow down on more carbohydrates calories than we need.

Just one cup of pasta, for example, contains 43 grams of carbohydrates. One measured cup is only the size of most people's cupped hand and adds up to almost half the total daily carbohydrate intake (of around 100 grams) that the average sedentary person looking to lose weight should consume.

Most people who sit down to eat pasta or grains (such as rice) eat a lot more than the size of their cupped hand. Usually a double serving fills half the typical dinner plate (around 86 grams of carbohydrates). If you go out to eat at an Italian restaurant for a cheap all-you-can-eat pasta night you are likely to consume a triple serving of pasta (129 grams of carbohydrates), plus all the extras such as the fats and calories in creamy sauces.

So, it's not the evil macronutrient magic of carbohydrates or the insulin fairy that makes you gain weight; it's the form they take that allows more calories to be consumed. That's not the kind of easy eating we want.

THE TWO RULES OF STARCHY CARBOHYDRATES

#1. Carbohydrates for Weight Loss: Did you Earn Them Today?

Like taking your car for a road trip and needing to refuel, if you burned up extra energy today exercising (especially resistance training) or were highly active for at least 30 minutes, then it's okay to choose a controlled portion of starchy carbohydrate or grain-based foods, like breads, pasta, potatoes, rice, beans or legumes in your meals that day. Why?

Because resistance training, and high intensity interval training especially, is fuelled by muscle glycogen (stored carbohydrate sugar in your muscles) that is used in short-burst activity like weight training and sprinting, your post-workout meal is the prime time to ingest higher carbohydrate foods as they will get pushed back into your muscle cells for energy replenishment and muscle recovery. Outside the post-workout meal, it's best to choose vegetables or fruits for your carbohydrates and keep your meals consisting of protein and produce.

Perfect Your Plate

Here are three real life *Easy Eating Diet* meal examples, first of a 'Protein and Produce' plate and second of a 'Protein and Produce Plus' plate, containing extra post-workout carbohydrates depending on when you had a workout.

Breakfast Protein and Produce Meal: Three-egg omelet with spinach, chopped peppers, onions and a little shredded cheese (thumb size). One half cup or (size of cupped hand) of fruit (like one apple, one orange or one serving of berries).

Breakfast Protein and Produce Plus Meal: Three-egg omelet with spinach, chopped peppers, onions and a little shredded cheese (thumb size). *Plus* one slice of toast with one serving of jam, or one half cup serving (size of cupped hand) of fried potatoes or one listed serving of oatmeal.

Lunch Protein and Produce Meal: Burrito Bowl containing shredded chicken or beef (palm size), spinach or lettuce, peppers, onions, salsa, and guacamole (thumb size).

Lunch Protein and Produce Plus Meal: Burrito Bowl containing shredded chicken or beef (palm size), spinach or lettuce, peppers, onions, salsa, and guacamole (thumb size) *plus* one half cup or (one cupped-hand serving) of added rice or beans. Or you can prepare the burrito bowl without the rice or beans and with the above protein produce ingredients, but wrap it instead in a flour or corn tortilla for extra post-workout carbohydrates.

Dinner Protein and Produce Meal: Palm-size serving of steak with one fist-size serving of roasted asparagus, broccoli, or green beans drizzled with 1 tbsp or (thumb size) of olive oil or melted butter.

Dinner Protein and Produce Plus Meal: Palm-size serving of steak with one fist-size serving of roasted asparagus or broccoli drizzled with 1 tbsp or (thumb size) of olive oil or melted butter, *plus* one-half cup (one cupped-hand serving) of rice, roasted potatoes or pasta.

If you don't want extra starchy carbohydrates post-workout, no problem. But I recommend you double your serving of fruit or vegetables to two fist-size servings of veggies or two pieces of fruit.

If you do choose starchy foods post-workout, unlike proteins and fats that fill you up almost automatically, portions need to be controlled as otherwise it's easy to overeat, overfill your tank of energy and offset the calories you burned through activity.

Obsessive meal math isn't needed, but if weight loss is your goal remember to keep a serving of starchy carbohydrates to the visual size of your cupped hand or measure out half a cup for a reference point, (just don't measure hot food in your hand!)

That amount in rice, pasta or potatoes contains approximately 25 grams of carbohydrates. Twenty-five grams of carbohydrates per meal is a good general guideline for how much carbohydrate intake is appropriate for those trying to obtain fat loss.

If you haven't done at least 30-minutes of good muscle-moving activity that made your heart rate go up and caused you to sweat, then chances are you simply didn't earn or burn enough energy to get away with consuming high amounts of carbohydrates from starchy grains, especially if fat loss is your goal. Those seeking to maximize muscle gain and high-performance activities always need more fuel.

So, the key thing to remember is that if you didn't exercise and burn some fuel stores and energy, only eat a fist-size serving of vegetables or one piece of fruit and you will still get lots of energy-rich nutrients, but without the excess carbohydrate calories.

If you are following a very low carbohydrate diet like Keto, don't forget that you are getting most of your energy from the fats in your foods and your body can even convert some protein into energy. But for *Easy Eating*, I like carbohydrates too much to lead you down that road.

> *The Easy Eating Diet is not anti-carbohydrate, low-carbohydrate or no-carbohydrate. It is a controlled*

carbohydrate approach to eating and the goal is to make eating easy again, so if you follow our recommended Smart about Starch System, you will get the best of both worlds by earning carbohydrates before you eat them and avoiding carbohydrates that disagree with your digestion.

This is where *The Easy Eating Diet* breaks away from the low-carb cult and 'Paleo Pack' and adds in science and common sense. If weight loss is not your primary goal and you are already lean or a high-performance athlete (performing high intensity exercise for more than an hour most days), you have higher nutrient needs and higher demands for carbohydrates and energy. If this is you, you will need to eat more carbohydrates to perform at that high level. So be sure to include some starchy carbohydrates in most of your meals to fuel your body and balance your plate along with additional *Easy Eating* foods.

Depending on your food preferences, and if grains is not your go-to, you can simply choose a double serving (the size of two fists) of fruits or vegetables instead of starchy carbohydrate-based grains and you will get plenty of energy for performance and recovery and a lot more nutrients per calorie. Yep, you can usually eat twice as much of mother nature's carbohydrates compared to man made carbohydrates!

Think about it. Nobody sits down and eats a bag of apples (mother nature's carbohydrates) but many of us can sit down and eat a bag of chips or crackers (man-made carbohydrates). So, don't fear fruit or carbohydrates from plants. Our obesity epidemic is certainly not caused by eating too much fruit.

Clearing the plate on the carbohydrate confusion boils down to this: the leaner and more active you are, the more carbohydrates and calories your body needs and can shuttle into your muscles to be burned as energy and not be stored as excess fat. Not there just yet? That's okay, as that's what this book is going to help you do.

#2 Carbohydrates for Health: Can You Digest Grains and Gluten?

Gluten is common in a lot of food. *The Easy Eating Diet* breaks free of diet dogma and bites into the popular gluten-free food trend. Gluten might be an issue for you, or it might not. Here's what you need to know.

You probably have heard enough about gluten over the last few years, but a quick de-brief about it is that it's a protein found in wheat and many grain-based products and it gives bread that gluey and gooey good texture and taste.

Unfortunately, according to celiac.org there is a very small percent of the population, around one percent, who have Celiac disease, a diagnosed autoimmune disorder or a complete gluten intolerance. These people are unable to digest and break down the gluten in foods properly. In them, the ingestion of gluten, a protein found in grains like wheat, rye, and barley, gives rise to antibodies that attack the small intestine.

At first, the symptoms are annoying: stomach aches, gas, and diarrhea. Over time, they can grow to be debilitating. The autoimmune assault corrodes the small intestine's ability to absorb nutrients, which can prompt anemia, chronic fatigue, and unhealthy weight loss. There is one treatment for Celiacs: strict, lifelong adherence to a diet that's devoid of gluten.

But there is also around five percent of the population (still not as big as the food marketers want us to believe) who have forms of non-celiac gluten sensitivity (NCGS). NCGS is not as 'black or white' in terms of diagnosis and it falls under a wider scale of symptoms that depend on the individual's tolerance level and can be escalated or improved depending on a person's health and lifestyle factors. As opposed to Celiac disease, where a sufferer must avoid gluten 100 percent of the time, gluten sensitivity is not as severe and small or occasional amounts of gluten can be tolerated, especially after improvements in gut health are made.

Here's my personal story about gluten and how discovering my sensitivity changed my life.

I was tested for gluten sensitivity in 2012 and discovered I had a high sensitivity to gluten. Eliminating it solved a life-long mystery of health issues. But prior to that, I discovered by accident that it was an issue for me.

With my passion for fitness, at age 21, I competed in my first bodybuilding contest. To prepare for competition I endured three months of strict dieting and ate the typical body-building diet foods of oatmeal, eggs, protein shakes, chicken breasts and vegetables.

Yep, literally; that's what I ate every day for three months to achieve the glorified 'ripped like a bag of milk' look we see in fitness magazines so that I could compete on stage. I didn't even put as much as a tic-tac into my mouth as I did not want to cheat on my diet. And naturally I didn't consume all the regular gluten-containing foods of breads, pasta and pizza.

I got into the magazine-type shape I always dreamed of and even appeared in a magazine, as I placed second in a worldwide body transformation contest. But after posing for the photo-shoot I immediately stuffed my face with a large pizza and chocolate cake (like every starving bodybuilding competitor does). And then I got to reflecting on this experience and all the intense training and dieting I did.

What I realized and didn't immediately notice due to the immense focus I'd had on my contest preparation was that for the first time since I was 12 years old I went three months without a migraine headache, without stabbing joint pain (despite training in the gym harder than ever) and with no brain fog or inability to focus (my mental focus was sharper than ever during this contest diet phase). As I was also a busy full-time college student with a part-time job at the local recreation center, this was surprising. I should have been wiped out.

For three months straight, I worked out every morning at five a.m., went to school from eight in the morning to three in the afternoon and worked at the recreation center from four in the afternoon to midnight. Obviously, I wasn't getting enough sleep, but my drive and diet were so focused that I pushed through it. Now I realize how important sleep is for health, happiness and hormones, which I will cover later in this book.

Ever since I was about 12 years old, I suffered from life-long debilitating migraines, as well as chronic colds, sore throats, cankers sores, bacterial infections and, throughout my teens and twenties, digestive issues (with too many doctor visits and antibiotic prescriptions to count, which only made things worse I was later to find out). I just seemed to catch every common and not-so-common cold and virus that was going around.

Today, of course, I realize how terrible growing up on a diet of 70 percent 'healthy whole grains' and gluten-containing foods like breads, pasta and grains was for me. Combined with constant cycles of antibiotics, it wrecked my gut health and hence my immune system was poor.

Stabbing joint pain from my fingers to feet would come and go, but I passed it off as the price to pay for years of heavy weight-lifting and bodybuilding in my teens and twenties.

The unexplained emotional irritability and inability to focus, though I was generally a happy, naturally calm guy, was harder to explain. What made it even more frustrating was that I was a hard-working health and fitness fanatic and had been so from 15 years of age, pumping iron, popping vitamins and supplements like candy and, at that time, eating and exercising better than most people my age or older—or so I thought, given my diet full of protein, grains and some fruits and vegetables.

So I made the rounds of doctors, but not one of the many I saw ever asked about my diet, mentioned the word gluten to me or sent me for food sensitivity testing.

My migraines got so bad that one day, while walking to the gym with my friend, we had to call an ambulance because a head-ache and nausea hit so hard it felt like I had been hit in the head with a bullet. I was then rushed to our national health science center where I remember lying on the floor of the bathroom in the dark, screaming in pain after power puking, while I waited for a brain scan appointment with a neurologist to see what was the problem.

Nothing abnormal showed up on the brain scan, so the only thing they could give me were migraine medications and antibiotics for infection. One doctor went as far to ask, "you seem to know more about nutrition and vitamins than I do, so what do you think could be causing these problems?"

The internet was in its infancy at the time and my, as well as most people's, awareness of gluten sensitivity was limited. Of course I continued to take the medications as it was the only way I knew to combat my migraines and I also kept taking the antibiotics to battle my constant health problems. These drugs were a large part of my diet during my growing years, but, as I found out later, they only made my underlying problem a lot worse.

I remember reaching my tipping point of constant health stress as a young muscle meathead who all-of-sudden was battling another strange infection—that of an embarrassing yeast infection in my mouth known as oral thrush. In me, thrush manifested as constant cracking at the corner of my mouth that wouldn't heal despite constant steroid creams and antibiotic medications.

With the internet and Google now available (though painfully slow via dial-up) I did what many of us do and searched for information online, which made my situation even worse. As most of us know now, Googling your symptoms is never a good idea and my search kept bringing me to the scary self-diagnosis of having a serious auto-immune disease—or even HIV! As a young married man with a baby girl at home, this caused me unbelievable stress that had me shaking during the day and lying awake all night.

My stress escalated to a breaking point one day at our local pharmacy. While standing at the pharmacy counter waiting for yet another prescription for the oral thrush yeast infection around my mouth, the pharmacist looked down at me from her high perch over her reading glasses, did a double take and, with a confused look (after reading the prescription), passed me many boxes of medications labeled for 'vaginal yeast infections!'

As an active young man, proud of my successful health and fitness regime, and known as the local fitness fanatic, I was totally humiliated. I was also frustrated. Why was I cursed with this condition?

However, desperate for relief, I took the boxes of pills and tumbled them discreetly into the noisy crumbled prescription bag they gave me, ran out to my car, sat there and finally broke down and cried hysterically.

"What the hell is wrong with me?" I raged, screaming to the heavens. I work so much harder than most at learning about and taking care of my health and fitness and it just doesn't make sense!"

It makes much more sense to me, after 24 years living and breathing everything health and fitness and working in the industry as a personal trainer and lifestyle coach. Now I know that 70 to 80 percent of our immune system is in our gut and digestive system. Destroy that, and add soul-sucking stress to the mix, and your health starts to crumble.

I've also learned not to Google health symptoms because it can send you into a scary rabbit-hole of unneeded panic and peril.

So, for those who have poor gut and digestive health, starchy carbohydrate-based foods like grains, beans and legumes that are commonly regarded as healthy, (because they are nutrient-dense in plant protein and fiber) might not be good for *you*, because they contain anti-nutrients like lectins and phytic acid, which are plant compounds that reduce the absorption of nutrients from the digestive system. This makes them hard to digest for some people.

My personal health dictates that I choose white rice over brown rice for this same reason; for me, it's easier to digest. The harder-to-digest grain, bean or legume is these plants' natural defense, as they don't want to get digested and destroyed; they want to stay intact so they can pass through your digestive system, be excreted and return to the earth to sprout and reproduce. The long-time practice of pre-soaking these foods can help them break down for easier digestion and assimilation, but this is not entirely effective.

It's a common tune about 'tooting': "Beans, beans the musical fruit, the more you eat the more you toot!" While a little blame-game office humor after lunch is common and even funny (to some), gastric distress should not be part of your life when you eat normal, healthy food. Certainly the uncomfortable gastric distress experienced by me and many others who can't tolerate heavy grains, beans and legumes should make you wonder if it's worth the pain. When we listen to our bodies, in the case of beans and legumes, the effects are easy to hear!

Again, despite those foods with anti-nutrients, we are not anti-anything with *The Easy Eating Diet*. Letting go of a little gas is a normal part of digestion, especially with high fiber plants and beans and legumes are nutrient-dense. But how food makes you feel after you eat it is something you need to think about. That's how you find the foods that are right for you. Because you don't have to eat beans and legumes when there are so many other options for consuming protein fiber and getting energy.

If you really enjoy beans and legumes, they give you no big issues and they are a common part of your food culture, no problem. Some of the longest-living cultures around the world have rice, beans and legumes in their diet, because they have evolved to adapt to this staple. I just personally leave them out of my diet and out of common recipes like chili, burritos and salads and instead I use other vegetables in their place to create a similar taste and texture.

BE GOOD TO YOUR GUT

With the recent rise of the popularity of probiotics (you probably have heard about these beneficial belly bacteria in the news), many of us now stock them on our supplement shelves and eat them in foods like yogurt, where they are commonly added during production. You would think that would make your belly dance around your kitchen in a crop top and grass skirt. But it doesn't work for all of us.

Our guts have within them both good and bad bacteria, but the constant pounding my gut took from my gluten sensitivity and subsequent cycles of antibiotics destroyed the good bacteria in my gut as well as the bad, which was not good for my health in the long term.

For me, being unaware of my gluten sensitivity and constantly ingesting and trying to digest high-gluten foods (that I ate a lot of growing up, as I am also a food fanatic who loves to cook and has a passion for all things pizza) led me to a tipping point.

As a young guy building my body up in the gym I could get away with pounding down all those carbohydrates and calories from an energy-burning point of view; but on the inside my body was breaking down. I thought the food sensitivity and health issues I was experiencing were just part of the process of eating huge amounts of calories to gain muscle size. I had yet to connect the dots.

Given my eating habits and the constant antibiotics, all the good bacteria in my gut meant to protect my immune system had been destroyed.

Picture the good bacteria in our gut as bouncers at a bar, stopping the trouble-makers and creeps from joining the party. Well, my bouncers were constantly getting beaten up and beaten down from the bad guys (bad bacteria) trying to get in, which was leaving the bar (my immune system) wide open, letting infections and intruders that normally would have been kept out of my bloodstream in to raise hell. This is also known as leaky gut syndrome.

I had one mysterious health issue after another and finally I got a bad C-difficile infection (C-difficile causes colitis by producing toxins that damage the lining of the colon). The symptoms of C. difficile are fever, diarrhea and abdominal pain, all of which I battled for a good month while trying to maintain a normal work and family life.

I also started to become allergic to apples for the first time in my life and they caused my lips to swell and a scratchy throat—this from a healthy food I always ate. Fresh cherries caused the same reaction on a few occasions. I discovered later that what I had was known as oral allergy syndrome and it was brought on by poor gut health. So much for 'an apple a day keeps the doctor a way!' Strawberries can be another common trigger for oral allergy syndrome for many people.

All this was a food fight I no longer wanted to be a part of. Only years later, when I discovered it was gluten creating this cascade of health symptoms and issues did I understand and connect the dots. After eliminating it from my diet, first via my bodybuilding training and then through an elimination diet, it became clear that all those frustrating health issues magically went away!

No more migraines, no more digestive upset, no more constant gas pains, no more joint pain, irrational irritability and brain fog. Plus, I got leaner and achieved and maintained visible abs without really trying and suffering through a strict bodybuilding contest diet to get them. Today, with better gut health, I still stay away from apples by simply eating other fruits I enjoy—but I can eat them cooked with no issues, as cooking breaks down the active proteins that cause reactions.

Gluten is not an issue for most people, but food sensitivities are real, for me and many others, and they can be especially escalated in those with poor gut health. So, if you experience any of the symptoms mentioned and you think you may have an issue with gluten, try an elimination diet where you don't eat foods containing gluten for 30 days. Note how you feel during and after the 30-day period then reintroduce the food into your diet and note any changes to how you feel physically and mentally. If you then want to dig further and get a more detailed assessment about your sensitivity level, get a food sensitivity test done by a doctor or local holistic practitioner. There are even home test kits available online from highly accredited labs around the world such as Cyrex or Entero Labs (which is what I used).

Over the years I have improved my gut health even more not just by the removal of these inflammatory foods but also by introducing supplemental probiotics, glutamine and fermented foods naturally high in probiotics into my diet, such as unpasteurized sauerkraut. One serving of sauerkraut has as much probiotics as an entire bottle of most probiotic supplements! With restored gut health, I can now even enjoy an occasional wheat crust pizza or gluten-containing food without any extreme adverse reactions. Sourdough bread made in the artesian way with a starter culture is especially tolerable as the fermentation process breaks down much of the gluten.

Being a pizza snob, I save my splurges for special occasions such as when I visit an authentic Italian restaurant where they serve Neapolitan style pizza cooked in 90 seconds in a wood-fired oven. Like me, many people find that food made with authentic Italian flours and baking methods that break down gluten through natural fermentation and bacterial cultures, affects their sensitivity and digestion less. Many believe it's because the wheat is less processed than GMO (Genetically Modified Organism) grown wheat. I believe it may be due to it not being sprayed with a common pesticide containing glycosphate which most modernized industrial wheat crops are sprayed with. Think about the weed killer you may spray on your lawn. Most of North America's commercial wheat crops are coated in this stuff!

CHAPTER 4:
DON'T FEAR FATS

As mentioned in the beginning of this book, we no longer need to fear natural fats in foods like we used to. We actually know now there are essential fatty acids like omega 3's that we need to consume to survive, not to mention thrive.

Our brain is made up of around 70 percent fat; further, our hormones, which are special chemical messengers in the body that are created in the endocrine glands and control most of our major bodily functions, from simple basic needs like hunger to complex systems like reproduction, and even our emotions and mood need healthy fats to be produced, balance and function properly. The trillions of cells in our body have an outer layer of fat around the cell membrane that needs to be comprised of those healthier fats to allow nutrients to flow in and out of cells efficiently and to put up a strong fight against the daily threat of disease.

Natural fats from animal-based foods, especially grass-fed meats, cold water fish, fish oils, plants, dairy, egg yolks, nuts and seeds all give us a variety of omega- 3, 6 and 9 fatty acids. Most of us simply need more anti-inflammatory omega-3's, found in natural foods, and less more inflammatory omega- 6 and 9's found in many processed foods and oils.

The most important omega-3 fatty acids are alpha-linolenic acid (ALA), eicosapentaenoic acid (EPA), and docosahexaenoic acid (DHA). Alpha-linolenic acid is an essential fatty acid: "essential," meaning that it must be provided in the diet or through supplementation. The body can convert ALA into EPA and DHA; however, the conversion is very inefficient, so dietary intake of EPA and DHA is important. EPA and DHA both play a crucial role in the development of the brain and central nervous system. in addition to their potent anti-inflammatory properties.

Since omega-3 and omega-6 fatty acids are a part of every cell in the body, changes in dietary composition of fatty acids has a direct effect on the concentration of fatty acids in your cell membranes. This in turn has an effect on the amount of inflammatory versus anti-inflammatory eicosanoids produced by your cells. Historically, the ratio of omega-6 to omega-3 in the diet was roughly 2:1; however, recently, an increase in the use of vegetable oils in the western diet has raised that ratio to as high as 20:1. The current recommendation to improve the omega-6 to omega-3 ratio is to increase the amount of omega-3 fatty acids in the diet. As you might suspect, reducing the amount of omega-6 (vegetable and seed oils) will also help to improve this ratio.

For fat consumption, cooking oils such as coconut oil, avocado oil and butter (grass-fed is preferred as it's higher in omega-3s and vitamin K2 than from grain-fed cows) are best for health and higher-heat cooking, as these fats have more health-promoting properties, are less refined and have higher smoke points (can withstand higher temperatures during cooking without breaking down).

Olive oil is great too, of course, but it is best for lower-temperature sautéing or baking, or for using in salad dressings, marinades or drizzling over food. Too high of a heat will break down the healthy benefits of olive oil.

I recommend you minimize all the other common vegetable oils, like canola, grapeseed, safflower and soybean oil etc., in your diet as they are highly processed and inflammatory.

CHAPTER 5:
THE 6 BEST FAT LOSS TRICKS AND TIPS

Below I've complied some of the best real-world fat loss tips I have learned over the last 24 years of health and fitness coaching.

1. Hack Hunger. Control your hunger and increase satiation without blowing your diet, especially on the weekends. This is the key to sustaining a diet and losing fat. Some people can white knuckle through the cravings without caving in to them, and some people don't have that kind of willpower.

But this is what separates the people who make consistent progress and those who don't. The weekends are when people struggle the most. Weekdays give us structure, but the weekend often means going out with friends or attending family functions. This is when you can blow your week's work of progress. A Saturday and Sunday of over eating/over drinking can undo the previous five days of being on plan with your diet, so you have to stop the self-sabotage if it happens to you.

2. Drink Diet. Drink a diet drink every time over a sugary soda. They're great at temporarily controlling your cravings and help you stay away from extremely high amounts of sugar calories—which is rock-solid proven to harm your health and contribute to obesity.

Again, no diet dogma here; believe what you wish but don't let the fear mongering about artificial sweeteners hold you back from an occasional diet soda. From all the research and reviews I have seen over the years there is no current evidence showing that regularly consuming a moderate amount of artificial sweeteners is harmful to your health. In fact, if artificial sweeteners can help you achieve a healthier body composition by taking the place of excess sugar and calories then it can be argued that they may help you become healthier. From all the smart minds in health and fitness I have personally met over the years, aside from the fact that they choose diet drinks over sugar-filled regular soda themselves, they also advise to choose low or no calorie drinks over sugary sodas or juices to lose or control your weight. Water, tea, or coffee is best, for sure. But still choose a diet drink over sugary soda when given the choice.

These days you can have the best of both worlds and get sugar-free soda like Zevia, that is naturally sweetened with stevia instead of aspartame or sucralose. Also, those home SodaStream machines are great for making your own sparkling water in seconds. You can get naturally flavored packs or liquid drops to flavor your water in flavors ranging from refreshing fruit punch to pink lemonade. Adding real berries or sliced lemon to water is another great flavor option. Again, just do everything you can to stay away from drinking regular soda and sugary drinks.

To also help hack hunger, load up on vegetables. Rich in fiber, veggies fill you up and you can eat a lot for little cost in carbohydrates and calories but a large benefit in nutrients. You'll never need to check into a weight loss clinic because of your broccoli habit. For easy eating at home, roast a big pan of any veggies you like tossed in olive oil and some spice and fill up on some produce with your protein.

If you're attending a get-together or event, bring a vegetable and deli meat tray and you can eat from it as you wish. Or if you are at an event and only sandwiches are supplied, you can take the deli meat off pre-made sandwiches (if there is no separate meat spread). This at least gives you a fighting chance at not ingesting a day's worth of carbohydrates in that baguette or ciabatta bread buffet.

Also having a scoop of whey protein shaken in water or a protein bar before leaving the house can curb your appetite big-time before you hit a function or eat out at a restaurant, and it'll minimize overeating.

3. Bite it and Write It, Drink it and Ink It. Also known as writing down everything you eat and drink into a food journal. If you have never done so before and are struggling with losing weight, track your daily calories and macronutrients (protein, carbohydrates, fats) for at least a week. Because if you are overweight, chances are your food portions are simply too big, leading you to eat too many calories and carbohydrates and not enough protein and healthy fats.

You need to get brutally honest with yourself about your diet and keeping an accurate food journal will show you and anyone helping you how the typical foods and meals you eat add up faster than you think in terms of calories—even some of the healthier foods you may be choosing can be higher in calories than you think. Journaling also allows you to see if your macronutrients, such as protein, carbohydrates and fats are in the proper balance for your health and weight loss goals. Remember, protein and fats are essential and you need a certain amount daily for health, muscle and metabolism. But for weight loss, at the end of the day all calories count, so assess, don't guess. You can then adjust portion sizes so as to hit your target fat loss numbers until your weight starts to drop in the range of one-half to one pound a week. Tracking can show you the difference between 'health' foods and 'fat-loss friendly' foods. Yeah, nuts are healthy, but if you're going nuts with them and taking in 500 extra calories a day by nibbling a handful of them, it'll be difficult to consistently get into that calorie deficit necessary for weight loss.

What you think is eating 'good' or 'healthy' may not be good enough to induce change in your body. If you aren't losing weight and are only hitting your target numbers 60 percent of the time, you need to bump that average up to 80 percent. Weight loss doesn't require meal math perfection but it does require discipline and consistency over time until you see or feel change in your body. One good or bad day of eating won't make a difference; it's the weeks and months that matter.

Sometimes subtle shifts are all that's necessary to start the fat loss process, or to keep it progressing. Some people jump to extremes when it's not necessary. Maybe all you need to do is to cut your calories or carbohydrates down by 10 percent daily to spark some fat loss, which boils down to removing a palm size portion of higher calorie food from your daily diet. Think along the lines of choosing some broccoli for bread and you are moving in the right direction.

By tracking, testing, and assessing, instead of going to extremes and cutting your calories too drastically, or cutting carbohydrates down to Keto style zero, you can learn an eating style that you can live with in the long-term.. If you like that style of eating and it works for your body and lifestyle, that's totally cool.

Food tracking, either using old school pen and paper or the many website and apps out there like MyFitnessPal, isn't something you need to do forever. The whole point is to teach you enough about nutrition so that you can eat more intuitively while still reaching your goals. You'll soon be able to make a good guess about the protein, carbohydrates and fats in a typical meal and will be able to eyeball or hand-size portions. Tracking is also good for those who just want to maintain; when 'diet creep' begins and you gradually start to slide off course, a few weeks of tracking can get you back on track again.

4. Improve Insulin. Insulin is a hormone that is normally released by the pancreas. Insulin sensitivity is how sensitive the body is to the effects of insulin. To be insulin sensitive will require smaller amounts of insulin to lower blood glucose levels than someone who has low sensitivity. Improving your body's insulin sensitivity might sound like a boring health tip from your doctor. But you really can improve your insulin sensitivity right away and at the same time help your body lose fat while you improve your health.

Remember, I said 'help your body lose fat,' not 'instantly erase 300 percent more body fat in the next hour' as some marketing madness might lead you to believe.

When you improve insulin sensitivity in your body, you can often eat more food without gaining weight. Insulin sensitivity determines how lean and toned you are. It improves the way your body partitions energy so that energy from the food you eat is preferentially shuttled to muscle instead of stored as fat. That's what I call the good grey zone of easy eating! It's why lean, fit people can eat more carbohydrates and calories than their heavier counterparts and still stay lean and fit.

If your insulin sensitivity is poor, you might look and feel squishy, or you might be reasonably lean everywhere except for a layer of excess fat around your waist. So you should incorporate as many of these insulin-sensitizing tricks as you can:

- Take two tablespoons of apple cider vinegar before bed or upon waking and/or use it in salad dressings and marinades. Taking it before a meal has been shown to improve post-meal insulin sensitivity by 30 to 40 percent.

- Sprinkle two to three teaspoons of cinnamon over your breakfast oatmeal, yogurt or shake. It slows down how fast your food digests and reduces fasting insulin levels.

- Take one teaspoon of psyllium husks twice a day (found in Metamucil) or find it as a solo ingredient in health food stores. Research demonstrates that using it for eight weeks reduce all-day blood sugar levels by 11 percent, plus it helps keep your bowels functioning properly.

- Take two servings of a high-quality omega-3 fish oil daily. Besides all the anti-inflammatory health benefits for brain, hormones and cells, fish oil also makes cells more sensitive to insulin and reduces secretion of insulin by the pancreas. It's one of the most natural health and metabolism boosters available.

There are two more things you can do too, but they have more to do with how you eat rather than what you eat or take with your food.

- **Chew Your Chow**. Try to be more mindful when you eat and take at least 15 minutes to eat your meal to allow proper digestion and ensure satiation hormones kick in to dampen any big spikes in insulin.

- **Prioritize Protein and Produce**. When sitting down to a meal, eat some protein or vegetables before you take even a bite of a starchy carbohydrate. Studies have shown this practice leads to significant reductions in post-meal blood sugar levels, simply by slowing down the digestion of those carbohydrates.

5. Protect Your Eating Environment. If you can't stop overeating a certain food, then you to need to keep it off your grocery list and don't bring it into your home, workplace, or car—because these are the places where you spend most of your time.

This tip may sound simple, but you can't eat what's not there, right? I have been saved from many food binges after a long stressful day because I searched for junk in my house but came up empty-handed because we keep it out of the house.

This period of going without your favorite snack is a great time to find alternatives that hit the spot. Do they have to be superfoods? No. You don't have to snack on raw broccoli or drink green juices to lose weight. But your food choices do need to be better than those you are currently making if you want to make changes to your body.

Make better 'choice trades' for what you are craving; for example, don't swap your bag of chips for crackers. Try snacking on something else that has the main flavor quality you're after. Is your favorite snack salty? Wrap a couple slices of deli meat around some cheese or smear some guacamole on a flavored rice cake and satisfy your salt craving that way.

Many nutrition 'gurus' will stick up their nose at these tips and say these aren't perfect superfood choices. For instance, rice cakes are a processed food and contain 'empty' calories they might say. But I say if those 35 empty calories (topped with another 100 calories of something else) can replace the 900 calories of what you were going to eat instead, it's a step in the right direction.

What if your favorite junk food is sweet? Find a sweet alternative. Mix chocolate protein powder with Greek yogurt and a tablespoon of chopped nuts or berries. Or consider a banana with a smear of peanut butter.

There are endless amounts of alternatives if you're creative enough and willing to try things. Yes, you need to try new things and make new choices. But go to the store and walk past the stuff you know you'll over-eat, because if you put it in your cart, it's going to end up in your mouth despite your best intentions. Make things easier, not harder for yourself.

6. Control Carbohydrates. Muscle tissue is the engine which burns dietary fuel (calories). Losing fat requires your body's engine to burn more calories than you ingest, forcing it to tap into stored calories (fat). The more lean muscle your body is composed of, the more calories you will burn. Eating too many carbohydrates makes it darn near impossible to get lean, as carbohydrates are just high energy that most people are not active enough to burn off.

At the same time, complete elimination of carbohydrates makes it difficult to function and work out for many and it is impractical for most people to do this. Therefore, the best way to lose fat is to replace starchy carbohydrates with produce-based carbohydrates obtained mostly from veggies and a little fruit. In addition to lean protein, ensure you also consume limited amounts of healthy fats (coconut, olive, avocado etc.).

7. Man or Woman Up. Time for some tough love. Stop thinking of food in terms of reward or punishment. Learn to cook and make healthy food taste good. Get off the strict start-and-stop diet train and find the middle of the road choices that bring progress and get you to where you want to go.

The solution is to simply choose better foods *most of the time*, not superfoods *all* the time and be consistent with some *exercise for a long time*. It's important to be consistent with exercise that appeals to you instead of being inspired for short periods of time with exercise you don't like.

You don't need a magic meal plan or an exercise machine that fits under your bed; you need to put into practice daily lifestyle habits of eating and exercise based on proven principles and allow for flexibility in your approach over time. Strive for progress, not perfection.

> *"Choose better foods most of the time, not superfoods all of the time, and be consistent with some exercise for a long time."*
>
> —Sean Barker

You also need to develop self-discipline and self-control. Planning meals and scheduling time for exercise isn't a bowl of fun but success in any endeavor requires the ability to get comfortable being a little uncomfortable in order to get a great reward. It wasn't too long ago that being disciplined and mentally strong was considered desirable traits. Where has that gone?

Like legendary strength coach and author of "Never Let Go" Dan John, says, "Eat like an adult. Stop eating fast food, stop eating kid's cereal, knock it off with all the sweets and comfort foods whenever your favorite show is on, ease up on the drinking and snacking and eat vegetables and fruits more. Stop with the whining. Stop with the excuses. Grow up."

We have to stop making excuses and take responsibility as grown adults no matter what the excuse. "But I have a busy work and family life that makes it hard for me to exercise and eat right!" you might say. Well, welcome to the real world. Excuses are usually regarding time, money or medical problems. But for every excuse I hear I see others with ten-times the obstacles getting results with their health and fitness.

I used to make the same excuses when I became a parent of one child, then two children and then I became a busy fitness business owner, speaker, writer, running multiple business ventures employing multiple employees, until I continued to see and meet fit parents running multiple bigger businesses and raising five kids, all while taking time for themselves to look after their bodies. The strong-willed person adjusts their diet and exercise to compensate for their back injury, thyroid problem or prescription medications. You have to be up for the challenge. You have to man or woman up and eliminate all excuses.

From, 'I'm big boned,' 'I'm too busy,' 'I can't afford a gym membership,' 'I don't know where to buy healthy foods.' to 'I don't know how to cook.' Remember, don't make things harder than they need to be. If you are currently doing nothing, doing something is progress. Start doing some body-weight pushups and squats most days and cook some meat and veggies in a pan for dinner and you'll be okay. Seriously, that's a great place to start.

Yes, I know it's not easy and that facing our excuses may hurt, but that's the only way real change is made. Doing anything worthwhile isn't easy. But this is *your* body, your health and happiness we are talking about! In today's world we are so busy and stressed, it's easy to get overweight, sick and tired. It's hard to lose weight and keep it off. It takes work. It takes planning. It takes discipline and determination. It takes reading books and asking for help from experts.

But like anything worthwhile, it *should* be hard in order to separate those who really want rewards and are willing to put in the work. It's what we teach our kids right? So let's listen to our own advice.

And one last thing: real results, real change will take *way* longer than you think. Longer than a few days, longer than a few weeks, longer than a few months. However long it takes, it's worth it. No eating or exercise tip will work until you remember that.

> *It will take longer than you think.*

CHAPTER 6:
WINE AND YOUR WEIGHT.

Alcohol in moderation can be a part of a healthy diet (full disclosure, it is a part of my diet). Like many people, I enjoy a good glass of wine with dinner, a cold beer on a hot summer's day or a drink of rum with friends. Even many of the longest-living cultures around the world have a little alcohol in their diet. If you don't drink alcohol, however, you certainly don't need to start.

Like anything you ingest, with alcohol, the poison is in the dose.

However, if you are unhappy with the way your body looks and feels and you drink frequently or binge on most weekends, you need to stop and think before you drink. Any source of liquid calories that you frequently consume is easy to over-consume and will make a big difference to your total daily calories.

To control your weight and your physical and emotional health, monitor what you drink and cut back if necessary. It's common to see people drinking a couple of 'glasses' of wine in glasses so big they can hold a whole bottle! This is not a good diet strategy. The easy calories from alcohol add sugars into the body and trigger the insulin response. Therefore, the more alcohol you drink, the more you will want to eat and it's usually not chicken breast and broccoli you will crave.

It's not just your palette that craves snacks high in fats, sweets and salt when you drink alcohol; to your body, alcohol is a toxin and once you ingest it, your body wants to consume the fastest sources of calories that it can in order to help absorb and balance the alcohol in your bloodstream. But all is not lost; if you want to enjoy alcohol in moderation and still achieve your best body you can follow the *Easy Eating* tip, below.

FOLLOW THE DRINK AND DINE 'FIT BODY FIVE'

When it's five o'clock somewhere remember that five ounces is one serving of wine (a little over the half-way mark in an average wine glass) and this serving clocks in at around five grams of carbohydrates and 120 calories. One 750 milliliter bottle of wine has approximately five servings and around 600 calories, with 25 grams of those calories being carbohydrates.

You can reduce your regular wine servings and accompanying calories by 50 percent by drinking only half a regular size glass at a time, or you can always make the choice to dietarily account for the carbohydrates in a full glass of wine at dinner by reducing or eliminating the starchy carbohydrates on your plate.

For beer drinkers, I always recommend light beer (at around 100 calories and six grams of carbohydrates per beer). With light beer, you can even afford a second one (if you must). However, if you choose regular beer (around 155 calories and 13 grams of carbohydrates) it's best to stop at just one, or reduce the calories of food you are going to eat in that meal or day to help compensate.

I always recommend naturally sugarless carbonated water or diet soda as mix in any hard liquor (around 86 calories per shot of spirits and zero carbohydrates). If you must choose a regular soda for mix (at around 150 calories and 40 grams of it sugar) it's best to stop at one drink. Whatever you choose, always go with the lowest calorie options because calories count (especially liquid ones) if you are working on your weight.

When making changes to comfort foods and drinking patterns in your everyday diet you may feel deprived of comfort at first, especially when it comes to sugar and alcohol, as they have strong biological and habit-holding effects. But discomfort isn't always a bad thing, and life without discomfort makes us unable to cope with common things that shouldn't be hard. Like avoiding the muffins at the office or making it to the gym.

To succeed in your weight loss goals, you must endure the unpleasant feelings that come along with changing your habits, especially at first. Train yourself to handle these feelings and they'll stop being unpleasant. Make small switches and swaps at first and eventually you'll look forward to all the better alternatives.

Big warning here: Avoiding drinks or foods you traditionally over-consume doesn't mean intentionally eliminating them 100 percent right away to slash your caloric intake drastically. That strategy will make you ravenous and more likely to overeat or drink later. Start by eliminating half the servings you normally consume, use simple swaps, try better alternatives and quit ignoring those sneaky eats and drinks that make you happy in the short term but overweight and unhappy later, sometimes for the rest of your life.

CHAPTER 7:
CALORIE CONTROL

Let's get one thing very clear – CALORIES matter **MOST** for WEIGHT loss.

I don't care what dietary protocol is popular that people are using—Keto, fasting, high protein, low carbohydrate, carbohydrate cycling, Weight Watchers, whole30, packaged meals, supplement shakes, or the many other diets that currently exist. There is no magic in any of them.

The magic is in the calorie control and finding the one you can follow consistently that will get you the results you want, and that you can maintain, without destroying your health.

It's crazy how so many people get up in arms and defend their favorite diet like a religious convert. Sorry to burst your bubble, but *all diets are just a way to control calories.*

Calories in versus calories out is still the rock-solid foundation of weight control, whether you're trying to lose or gain. I'm not sure when we thought we could start ignoring the irrefutable laws of thermodynamics, but we can't—period.

Sure, there are health and hormone benefits to different approaches, but I am talking about pure weight loss.

However, within the framework of 'calories in versus calories out,' there are a few considerations that still need to be made.

Although **the QUANTITY of the food (calories) you eat determines your body weight, the QUALITY of the food you eat (nutrients) along with your exercise determines the type of weight you will gain or lose and what your body fat percentage and total body leanness will be.**

Many people have proven the scientific fact that weight loss is always determined by caloric intake by following extreme diets of just fast food, supplement shakes, juicing, removing one food group or even just eating one food—anything from Twinkies to potatoes.

These types of extremes are not something any health professional would recommend, but they work every time to prove the point about 'calories in, calories out' for pure weight loss (as opposed to eating for just health and nutrition), because at the end of the day they put the body in a caloric deficit with weight loss as the the result. But we don't want you to sacrifice your health and happiness just to see a lower number on the scale. There are better ways to lose weight.

> "Calorie Quantity is King, Calorie Quality is Queen"

Five hundred calories of broccoli and 500 calories of potato chips, due to the difference in nutrient density and volume of food, will have vastly different effects on your body's energy levels, blood sugar, health and hunger hormones. Nutrients from broccoli will satiate the body, making long-term adherence to, and weight loss results from, that diet choice of chips very hard to maintain. That's why it's not so cut and dry as just cutting calories; both quantity and quality of food have to be considered in context.

Also, drastically lowering calories too much, too fast for faster weight loss is not better for you or healthy. It's true that yes, being in a caloric deficit is 100 percent required to lose weight. However, it is not true that the larger the deficit, the more weight will be lost. This is the biggest mistake people make when they try to lower their calories too much.

People who want weight loss fast and try to make the process even faster will benefit from a fast water weight loss at first (not fat loss) then hit a plateau that will make them feel "hangry" (hunger-induced anger) as hell most of the time. They will also lose lean muscle mass and—if they keep it up—develop horrendous health consequences, with weight rebounding back and no room to adjust caloric intake for long term maintenance.

So regarding calories, remember: **losing weight requires a calorie deficit.** However, most (not all) of the foods you eat still need to be nutritious. Small changes are preferred to drastic, large ones; dropping approximately 250 to 500 calories from your daily diet on average is key to long-term weight loss.

Basically, to give you a good visual, think of a palm-size of food reduction of food each day, or make a lower calorie food swap such as subbing spaghetti squash for pasta, or substitute greens for grains such as a meal with roasted asparagus instead of rice. Subtract another 200 to 500 calories burned through exercise a few days a week and you are in the zone.

NEED FOR NUTRIENTS

The studies that have been conducted on nutrition and weight loss are all relatively clear about a few things when it comes to macronutrients (protein, carbohydrates and fats).

First, daily caloric intake need to be set based on your current body composition, your activity levels and future goals. Your appropriate percentages of protein, carbohydrates and fat should be built and balanced on that, as should your calorie needs.

Second, after setting daily calorie goals, the next most important macronutrient to set up and control is protein. All research continues to show the two constants that need to be controlled for weight loss are #1 calories (caloric deficit), #2 protein (getting enough).

HOW MUCH PROTEIN PER DAY? HERE'S A GOOD GUIDE.

- **Take your DESIRED bodyweight GOAL and times it by .8.** For example, if you want to be 150lbs the formula is: 150X.8 = 120 grams of protein required daily.

- Based on the outcome of the formula above (in this case 120) eat 120 grams of protein per day. If you exercise most days of the week, do not go lower than 100 grams. If you are not eating that much protein right now that may seem like a lot of protein. But not enough protein in your diet is why you are probably struggling to get leaner and lighter and battling food cravings for sweets, salt and starches in the evening. Sound familiar? More protein is the answer almost every time.

Adequate protein is what works to get lean and it's how lean fit people eat. What it looks like is three good palm-size portions of protein-based food in a whole day, with an average palm full being 25 grams of protein (like one small chicken breast), one scoop of protein powder, a three-egg omelet with cheese or a small piece of meat or fish. Add a simple super shake to those three meals and you now have at least 100 grams of protein a day, easy-peasy.

As for carbohydrates and fats, no matter what the current diet and marketing madness says, you get to adjust the balance of carbohydrates and fats in your diet that suits your lifestyle and activity levels. Yay!

Do you like eating more carbohydrates? No problem, just eat a little less fat (that's how most ripped fitness competitors still eat since Arnold Schwarzenegger starred in *Pumping Iron* back in the 70s) and it's obvious that it works.

Do you like eating more fats instead of more carbohydrates? No problem, try to get most of them from omega-3 healthy fats and eat less carbohydrates instead (that's how the Keto no-carbohydrate diet works for weight loss too).

It's calories from the combination of fatty and high-carbohydrate convenience foods that pile on the weight fast. Foods like doughnuts, muffins, burgers with buns, French fries, pizza, ice cream and the cream and sugar in your coffee all add up. All these foods are carbohydrate AND fat bombs. They are yummy foods, but try having them as treat foods once a week, not once a day.

Science tells us that, taken separately, neither carbohydrates nor fats is more important when it comes to weight control. According to the EBioMedicine 2017 research review , Howell, S. and Kones, R. revealed the following conclusion in their recent study on calories and macronutrient balance:

"Strong data indicates that energy balance is not materially changed during caloric substitution of dietary fats or carbohydrates.

"Results from a number of sources refute both the theory and effectiveness of the carbohydrate-insulin hypothesis. Instead, risk for obesity and weight control is primarily determined by total caloric intake."

These statements tell us a few things: First, they reaffirm the notion that calories are the most important thing to consider during weight loss.

Second, they reaffirm that carbohydrates alone don't necessarily make you fat.

Third, they reveal that carbohydrate and fat distribution beyond calories-in and protein consumption are individual choices.

As for protein, you just can't skimp or make trade-offs as protein is essential to health, muscle and metabolism for so many reasons.

EVERYTHING ELSE

At this point, we have covered the two fundamentals that EVERY dietary protocol should be built upon. This includes every popular dietary trend you are *currently* hearing about from Keto to intermittent fasting and from carbohydrate cycling to Paleo. No matter the 'diet,' calories must be controlled and macronutrients must be properly set up based on those calories to meet the goals of the INDIVIDUAL. That's the key; you have to eat for *you*. Not for your spouse, your teenage son or your skinny friend. You need to eat for YOU and your goals.

> "Comparison is the thief of joy."
>
> — Theodore Roosevelt, 26th American President

CHAPTER 8:
ASSESS DON'T GUESS

How many calories do you need daily to begin your new, individual eating plan? You can eventually adjust, but you need to start somewhere. It's simple to figure out. Here is a guide to start with and always refer to.

- **Have you stayed the same weight over the last two weeks?** If so you are eating enough calories to maintain your current body weight.

- **Have you gained weight over the last two weeks?** If so, you are eating more calories than you need.

- **Have you lost weight over the last two weeks?** If so, you are in a caloric deficit. (one-half to two pounds a week is a safe average weight loss).

Other body composition tracking measures are also important for a clear picture of your current state, such as body fat percentage and inches. It's useful to measure around your chest, arm, waist, hips and thighs; but to set your daily diet calories, assessing your body weight is easiest.

Then **take your current body weight and times it by 12 to get your starting daily calorie range.** With that in mind, here is very clear action steps:

1. **Set it Don't Forget It.** Set your daily calorie intake relative to your goals, remembering to not be extreme in either direction. **Take your goal weight X 12 to start and if you have more ambitious goals, take your GOAL weight X 12.** Assess and adjust your calories up or down after two weeks. Yes give it at least 2 weeks!

   For example, a goal of 150 pounds X 12= 1800 calories daily. Start here then assess your progress every two weeks and adjust calories up or down until you see change.

2. **Prefer Protein.** Get enough daily protein. **Multiply your goal weight X .8**. For example, a goal of 150 pounds = 120 grams of protein required daily. Assess progress every two weeks and adjust only slightly.

3. **Pick Your Preference.** Choose your balance of **carbohydrates and fats based on your preference, exercise and activity goals**. More active people need more carbohydrates in their diet. Leaner people can eat more carbohydrates because they have more lean muscle to burn them off. So, if you are not there, it's a good place to be, so let's get there!

4. **Endure and Enjoy.** Remember, any changes you make from a dietary perspective should allow you to maximize your lifestyle. They should not feel like a strict diet or death sentence. **It takes work, but enjoy the ride** ok?

CHAPTER 9:
FASTER FAT LOSS

Let's break down fat loss into its three most important components:

1. Create a Caloric Deficit. Without a caloric deficit (consuming slightly less calories than your body needs to maintain your current body weight), you'll never lose fat, period. The easiest way to reduce your calories is by controlling what you eat. Burn some calories with exercise to slim and shape your body, absolutely! But even the most gruelling workouts burn just 300 to 500 calories an hour. In fast food land, that's just one typical small hamburger to erase all that hard work. Sad, I know. But that's the reality we are working with.

To shift your body into fat burning mode, your metabolism must burn more calories than you consume each day. How do you boost your metabolism and feed your metabolic machine? By consistently eating plenty of lean protein and vegetables at each meal, adding a little healthy fat and controlling carbohydrates. Want the easiest and most effective diet tip ever? Hold up your hand and make a fist. Now use this portable portion device that is specifically customized for your body type; yep your hand.

Make portion control simple when you start and don't eat any portions of protein, produce, and starch on your plate that are bigger than your fist. Is it perfect and precise? No. But it works, and it's a strong visual guide you can use anywhere to get you started to reducing calories without obsessing over the numbers and that's not complicated. It's also one that you will have 'on hand' at home, work or whenever you go out to eat to control calories when plated portions are double and triple than standard servings. Plus doing a fist pump before you eat is a little reminder to yourself, "I am strong, I got this!"

Eventually and especially if you are a small framed person looking to lose weight you may have to adjust your portions down to palm-size for protein, produce and starch for a simple switch that reduces the calories just a little more.

This one rule will be easy and effective for achieving your best body. That's as complicated as nutrition needs to be to get started and start seeing results, it really is. You select foods you like under the macronutrient categories of protein, produce and starch based foods, ensure variety so you don't get bored and use your hand as a calorie calculator. Refreshing eh?

2. Increase the Caloric Burn Through Exercise. In addition to managing portions and calories, you must also create a metabolic disturbance through challenging exercise that combines weight training and cardio. Exercise builds strength, burns calories (but remember it's small compared to food control) and boosts your resting metabolism long after your workout.

In terms of metabolic demand, there's a massive difference between a squat and an arm curl. The former challenges hundreds of muscle groups and stimulates your energy systems; the latter moves one single muscle the size of a baseball. Squats, pushups, pull-ups, burpees and deadlifts are some of the hardest but most effective exercises because they have a very high metabolic cost. Single joint exercises, or machine-based exercises where you're sitting, don't. Just make sure you learn how to perform them well from a good trainer.

3. Surround Yourself with Social Support. Is your boss forcing you to eat doughnuts at each meeting? Quit your job. Are your kids kicking and screaming for you to stop at the drive-thru on the way home? Give them up for adoption. Does your spouse have the pizza deliveryman on speed dial? Get a divorce! (KIDDING on all these of course) but you get the idea.

Without a doubt, one of the most difficult things about losing fat is eating in social situations. The peer pressure is the toughest test of your commitment. But if you want to succeed, you need to lay some ground rules. The days of excuses and blaming others or your surroundings are over; it's time to take back control. There is no room for debate. You are either in control of your eating and exercise decisions or you are letting others control you. And you might just surprise some folks when you show them that life can go on if you don't drink a whole bottle of wine or eat enough chicken wings to fly home after work.

So be loud and proud about what you are doing! There are more folks secretly wishing someone will take charge and be a healthy role model for them than there are wanting to see another person fail. It might not happen overnight, but if you continue to lead by a healthy example—without preaching or being condescending—you can build an entourage of social support and people who want to be healthy like you. This will build powerful support and relationships that will take your health to the next level.

If you don't create an environment that's conducive to losing fat and being healthy, you'll have a hell of a time losing your midsection and sticking around for many years to enjoy an active lifestyle with your family.

Remember, you are in the driver's seat and you need to put your foot down to move forward; the direction and guidance in this book is your GPS, showing you the proper eating and exercise strategies to guide you and get you back on track if you start to drift off course. Stay focused on your goals and don't give any time to those who try to sabotage your efforts.

Also, it is important not to let yourself get overwhelmed. There's no reason to. You have the tools to succeed.

> "Control what you can, cope with what you can't, and concentrate on what counts."
>
> —Craig Ballantyne, Author of The Perfect Day Formula

CHAPTER 10:
FIT BODY FANTASTIC FOUR RULES OF FAT LOSS

1. Do at least FOUR 30-minute workouts a week. Build up to it (if you need to) by starting with five-minute rounds of performing five different bodyweight exercises for 30 seconds of work each with 30 seconds of rest in between. One round through the five exercises is five minutes of on and off work, four total rounds is a 20-minute circuit.

I call this one '*The 30-30 Total Body Weight Blast*' workout, up to four rounds through each of the exercises A-E:

A. **Pushups:** Place your palms on the floor underneath your chest and shoulders. Beginners, place your knees on the floor behind your hips. Advanced, place your toes on the floor and brace your abdominals to keep your body straight from head to heels. Lower your chest to the floor and push up to lockout your upper arms.

B. **Squats:** With your feet hip width apart and toes pointed slightly out. Beginners, place your hands together in front of your chest (prayer style). Advanced, place your hands behind your head (prisoner style). Push your hips back and bend your knees but keep them from going in front of your toes. Lower down as far as comfortable (preferably until your thighs are level with your hips or legs 90 degrees, all while keeping your heels on the floor.

C. **Jumping Jacks:** Beginners, step out to the side, pushing your hip back and bend at the knee into a side lunge as you keep your opposite leg planted on the floor, then bring your hands together above your head. Alternate from side to side. Advanced, start standing with your hands down by your sides and feet together, and jump out to the side with your legs and bring your hands together overhead at the same time. Keep a soft bend in your knees and stay light on the balls of your feet as you jump in and out.

D. **Front Planks:** Similar to pushup progressions, except you place your forearms on the floor instead of your palms, hold your arms L-shape with your elbows underneath your shoulders and squeezing your fists. Beginners, place your knees on the floor behind your hips, brace your abdominals and hold for time. Advanced, place your toes on the floor with your legs straight, brace your abdominals, and squeeze your legs and butt cheeks tight to keep your body straight from head to heals and hold for time.

E. **Burpees:** In a squat stance, beginners, squat down until your hands are on the floor in front of you and step back one leg at a time into a pushup position with your body forming a straight line head to heels. Move one foot forward one leg at a time and stand up and reach your arms overhead. Advanced, squat down until your hands are on the floor, kick back both legs behind you at the same time while bracing your abdominals and locking your legs tight. Lower down into a full pushup and pushup back up and jump forward with both legs and jump up reaching arms overhead.

2. Eat FOUR times per day (three meals and one snack or shake)

3. Eat every FOUR hours during the day of those meals (three meals and one snack or shake)

4. Engage in FOUR hours of total activity a week.

(In addition to your four structured workouts a week, you will still need to move your body as much as possible).

That's it. Keep it simple and save your energy for your exercise instead of analyzing every small detail about how you are living and eating. Simply stay on track by asking yourself this one question at the end of every day or week:

"Did I follow the Fit Body Fantastic Four Rules of Fat Loss?"

If you answer yes six days out of seven, that's impressive and you are on the fast track to fat loss success. If you answered yes five days out of seven, that's great and you can still get impressive results. If you answered yes four days out of seven, that's good too, just not as great. Any less and results will take longer.

Work up to your best compliance and consistency and focus on improving on the one fat loss rule that you struggle with the most. You don't need perfection, just progress. Like everything in life, the '80-20 rule' will get you there: strive to follow these rules 80 percent of the time and the other 20 percent of the time you will have wiggle room for real life and pure enjoyment.

Remember, knowledge isn't power, it's just potential. Applied knowledge is power. The information in this book won't do you any good without steadfast implementation. However, you need to start somewhere and it's best to build up slowly if you wish to create sustainable lifestyle habits that you will stick with and results that will be permanent.

CHAPTER 11:
PRACTICE MAKES PROGRESS

Eating better to lose weight and feel great doesn't come from following a diet or eating based on a magic meal plan (you know, the one that everyone keeps looking for—you can find a million free ones on the internet). Again, it's not the information, it's the implementation.

If it was as easy as following the latest fad, we wouldn't be as heavy as we are. Magic diets are not the answer. **PRACTICE and PATIENCE are the answer**, because progress doesn't just happen and good behavior doesn't just become a habit unless you practice; and if you're practicing, then you are striving for progress not perfection.

Think about it: anything you learn in your life you need to practice and work at consistently to get better at. The same applies to getting in shape. You need to practice exercising in order to move better, build and shape your body. You don't attempt to lift 200 pounds on your first day in the gym because it takes trained skill, not will.

Eating better, like exercise, is also a PRACTICE. You shouldn't go into the kitchen on your first day of improving your diet and try to follow a strict meal plan diet of extreme food choices and caloric restriction ... because it takes trained skill, not will.

That's why *The Easy Eating Diet* is built around simple science and food foundations that give you structure—and also recipes—so you can customize your lifestyle and be flexible in what you eat.. There's no cheating the practice without putting in the 'reps' (repetitions) in losing weight or anywhere else in life.

Do you walk out of class in college the first time it gets tough? I hope not. The same applies to music or sports. If you want to be a musician, you practice guitar and piano. When you hit the wrong key on the piano or the wrong fret on your guitar do you throw in the towel for the day because you messed it all up, or your fingers are sore? No way! If you drop the ball someone passes you, do you walk off the field and give up?

It sounds ridiculous when we think about it that way, yet we do that with our eating plans and habits. We eat one cookie that's not on the diet plan and we think, 'I blew it, so I might as well go back to my normal routine of eating junk and maybe I'll try again on Monday.' As adults, we do that with food, but we'd never tell our kids to stop practicing piano because they hit a wrong note.

Start thinking that eating better food is just like any other practice because whether you want to or not, you practice eating every single day, so you might as well practice *good* eating habits. What you practice, you get really good at over time.

If you practice not eating everything on your plate, stopping when you are satisfied and not stuffed, you will get really good at it. If you practice not eating immediately when you feel little tummy tingles, or are stressed or sad, you will get really good at it. If you practice measuring proper portions and servings, you get really good at knowing how much is enough. And if you practice cooking healthier foods and learning simple recipes in the kitchen you will get really good at that!

So consider this—every time you eat, you are practicing.

Here are some important truths you must remember if you are going to make REAL LASTING CHANGE.

It's not going to be easy, and a lot of times you are going to practice what you think you already know. You may think it's too easy and that what you're doing doesn't matter or is not giving you rapid results. But it will give you results if you keep trying.

On the other end of the spectrum, maybe you are an all-or-nothing exerciser or eater, something I see with many of my clients. This type of person is perfect throughout the week but falls off the wagon on the weekends or when they travel. As soon as they slip up, they throw in the towel for the rest of the week then use their indescretion to binge and make big plans to start again the following Monday. Why do you have to wait until Monday to start over? Why don't you get back on track the very next day or even better, the very next meal?

Man, I see that all too often! Your body don't know what day of the week it is, it's all in your mind. That is just a vicious cycle of spinning your wheels and staying stuck.

If you are not the, 'eat one piece of dark chocolate after dinner' kind of person and are more of a, 'destroy a tub of ice cream if I'm going to have dessert' kind of person, you need to start PRACTICING becoming better and learn to eat a little less of what you want if you ever want to break the cycle.

Yes, it will be hard at first; but again, like playing guitar or exercising, you have to get comfortable being uncomfortable at first and then put in the practice and repetitions. With time and practice you will get better and soon will be able to have a little bit of dessert after dinner without going crazy with binges on the weekends anymore.

At times you will want to give up because it will be challenging. Don't.

Trust me it will become easy if you stay the course and put in the repetition. Changing habits may seem weird at first because you have been eating every single day of your whole life and you know how to do it; but in the same way that you can't just pick up a guitar and master Stairway to Heaven on your first attempt, you're not going to be able to master new ways of eating on your first attempt, and that's totally okay.

"Focus on progress not perfection."

— Bill Phillips, Body for Life Author

CHAPTER 12:
EASY EATING MEALS IN MINUTES

For breakfast, a favorite of mine, and a meal that works well for many clients, is old-fashioned oats covered with water and microwaved for one minute, then with one scoop of chocolate whey protein powder and one teaspoon of natural peanut butter added, stirred to combine.

Or to switch it up, use vanilla whey protein powder in the oatmeal and top it with blueberries, a sprinkle of hemp hearts and cinnamon and you have a breakfast that is high-protein, with fiber-rich carbohydrates and some healthy fat, all in a tasty, easy to eat breakfast in one minute.

Easy eating is especially what you want in the morning when you have one eye open and need to remove decision fatigue and rely on routine to get out the door and on with your day. I have also used this meal of protein oatmeal (or ProOats as I call it), as a last resort nutritious meal replacement for lunch or dinner on those crazy, busy days.

You can even put a healthy hack on something as simple as a bowl of cereal, though be careful with your cereal choice; breakfast cereal is far from being a superfood and most cereals found on the supermarket shelves are just processed boxes of sugar. As far as cereal goes, a listed one-cup serving of an old school classic like multi-grain Cheerios is just 110 calories, 24 grams of carbohydrates and, at 6 grams of sugar, one of the lowest content cereals for calories and sugar. You can get a big nutrient boost if you halve the serving of the man-made carbohydrate of cereal and double up on Mother Nature's carbohydrates. Fill up on such fruit as blueberries, a true superfood.

Most people eat a double serving of cereal (or more) then throw a few berries on top with a splash of milk. But by simply reducing your one-cup serving of cereal to one-half a cup and doubling up on blueberries (from one-half a cup to 1 cup), you reduce the starchy carbohydrates in your meal and greatly increase the fiber and antioxidants. As you enjoy your cereal (and lose the weight!), you can give the finger to those nutrition gurus who cringe at anyone eating such a carbohydrate-laden convenience food.

Do you want to give your bowl of cereal more protein power? Instead of just milk, get a shaker bottle and shake up a scoop of vanilla flavored whey protein in water and pour it over your cereal—and now you have 25 grams of protein instead of just 8 to 10 grams from the milk. Little changes like this that focus on better and not always best, makes a big difference and are how you build easy eating habits into the context of your real life for real results.

Of course, any way you like to whip up some of nature's perfect protein, eggs, is a good way. Eggs can be boiled, fried, scrambled or flipped as an omelet with some spinach, cheese or chopped veggies and it takes under ten minutes to prepare a tasty dish. And don't worry about the cholesterol content of yolks. That stigma has been debunked for years with it now commonly accepted that whole eggs are health-promoting. Yolks contain protein as well as essential fats and nutrients that can actually help reduce blood serum cholesterol.

Remember, an egg is designed with everything in it to nourish a growing life, so we need to stop messing with Mother Nature's recipes. Plus, you can always use a combination of liquid egg whites for convenience then throw in a whole egg or two to get the best of both worlds; super nutrients and calorie control.

Plain Greek yogurt or cottage cheese with mixed berries and cinnamon is also a great source of protein. Combine these things with produce and you have another simple meal in minutes. Watch the flavored yogurt with fake fruit, though, as this stuff can pack as much sugar as a candy bar.

At lunch, when you are on a tight schedule and away from home, finding filling food in sensible portions that doesn't bog your body down and have you crashing into a coma by afternoon is important. One of my healthy habits is simply to cook extra for dinner then take those leftovers for lunch. Try to always make extra when you cook, as it doesn't require much extra effort to have two frying pans or two baking sheets full of protein and produce cooking away at the same time.

Or even go old school and brown bag your lunch. Bring a turkey sandwich on some good-quality bread with lettuce and tomato, Dijon mustard and a small apple on the side— a decent meal choice containing protein, produce, and fiber-rich carbohydrates that will keep your calories in check and only takes minutes to make. Again, I bet some nutrition guru's eyes will roll at that recommendation. But the many clients I have helped who have lost weight and gained health through little changes like this wouldn't.

For dinner, planning goes a long way after a long day. If you plan your weekday dinner meals on a Sunday night, that's great. If not, shorter-term planning is still better than no planning, so decide the night before at least what meat or protein you are going have for dinner the next day and then take the ingredients out of the freezer (or better yet, have it fresh in the fridge).

Once you have your protein ready, all you need to do is decide what pairing of produce and/or starch to have with it. Following recipes is great, but only if you keep them simple, especially if you are crunched for time during busy weekdays and have a family to feed. Save the gourmet cooking attempts for the weekends, a special dinner party or a day off.

If you are fortunate enough to be able to outsource your diet to a meal preparation service then by all means use such a service. The modern conveniences available to us today are amazing; so use them.

Learning to cook and enjoy food with family and friends is a skill everyone should have, at least at a basic level. Over the last 20 years I have learned many cooking skills just from watching cooking shows and the Food Network. Having a cooking show on in the background while I cook inspires and educates me. Whatever works, do it. Because we gotta eat.

As a parent, one of the most valuable skills we can teach our kids is how to cook, the earlier the better. Many teenagers today don't know what half the foods are in the produce isle. Purple is a color, not a flavor. So get your kids into the grocery store and kitchen with you, teach them what real food is and don't be afraid to get messy. You will create memories to last a lifetime and give them the best skill, gift and chance to make eating easy and enjoyable.

There is no such thing as a magic meal plan or recipe but here's a sample **Easy Eating Meal Plan** to give you an idea.

Breakfast, Easy Eggs: Three eggs scrambled and mixed with a palm full of baby spinach and a thumb-size serving of cheddar-cheese. Ten-minute meal.

Snack Supershake: One scoop of vanilla whey or plant based protein powder in ice water, one cupped palm size or one-half a cup of frozen blueberries, one thumb-size (or 1 tablespoon of natural peanut butter), blended. One-minute meal.

Lunch, Superfood Salad: (bowl full of romaine lettuce, tomatoes, cucumbers) with one diced chicken breast, drizzled with a thumb-size (or 1 tablespoon) each of extra virgin olive oil and apple cider vinegar. With leftover chicken, a five-minute meal.

Dinner: Any beef, pork, fish, chicken or plant protein source portioned into the size of your palm, one cupped hand (or half a cup of rice), a fist-size serving of green beans with one thumb-sized serving of butter melted over them. 30-minute meal at most.

Other meal and snack ideas that don't involve complicated recipes:

- Cooked ground beef topped with spinach and salsa or with broccoli and extra virgin olive oil, bacon or sausage with cheese, and one-half a grapefruit on the side.

- Chocolate protein shake with ground flaxseed and frozen strawberries.

- Roasted chicken breast with spinach (wilt the spinach in a pan with minced garlic and extra virgin olive oil) and a small apple.

- Extra-lean ground turkey sautéed with peppers and onions.

- Roasted salmon (spread Dijon mustard on top before roasting) with mashed cauliflower or green beans. Choose the foods you like and the ideas are endless. That's *Easy Eating*!

CHAPTER 13:
THE THREE P'S OF PROGRESS: PROTEIN, PORTIONS, PLANNING

Progress. There is nothing more motivating when making positive changes and creating a healthier lifestyle than seeing results fast. We all want results *yesterday* and with the least effort possible. That's human nature but it's also the sneaky secret weight loss companies depend on for selling every weight loss diet, supplement or gadget. These types of results are short-lived, though, and the weight loss is usually short-term water loss caused by severe carbohydrate and caloric restriction. Also, if you don't stick to the magical plan (buy more of it), the weight rebounds back once you go back to your normal habits.

These diet plans are like the latest celebrity endorsed detox juice cleanse, or the magic exercise machine that can fit under your bed—they don't stand the test of time. Sorry to burst your bubble, but there are many men and women behind the big curtain at those companies trying to trick you into pulling out your wallet, which is the only thing that gets lighter when you chase the next false fix.

If you want real results, real progress that lasts for life, you have to adopt a 'slow and steady wins the race' approach and think about the bigger picture expecting smaller results over time. Expect to take at least 12 months to reach your goal, not 12 days.

1. Protein. We already covered protein extensively in this book so I won't say much more except that you know it must be important when every new diet or diet product (such as supplement shakes) still makes it a priority. There's been trends over the years toward high carbohydrate, low fat, high protein and high fat. But if you see a low protein diet, back away from that book! Because it's simply non-negotiable to decrease protein in a healthy diet if you want to be leaner and lighter and free from craving carbohydrates like the cookie monster.

2. Portions. We have also covered how portion control is mandatory to control calories if you want to control your weight. The easiest way to reduce calories without counting them with a calculator is by controlling the portions on your plate and in your daily diet. Eating proper portions of protein, produce and smart starch for YOUR calorie needs, body size and body-shaping goals will get you more progress than anything else.

3. Planning. Prepare to plan or prepare to fail—a lot. Remove decision fatigue and temptations as much as possible. If you just 'wing' your diet, you will end up eating wings.

CHAPTER 14:
SUGAR SHOCKER

Let's tip over another scared cow on the food farm. It may come as a bit of a shock after all you have heard in the media about nutrition, but sugar itself, in our food, (although more abundant than ever and like anything in excess can cause health issues) will not make you fat. Sugar is not the single biggest cause of obesity though sugar intake should definitely be controlled (especially if you are diabetic).

Like any other food, the only way you'll gain weight from eating sugar is if you consume too many calories of it. Look up any well-designed study controlling calories and you'll find that sugar does not cause weight gain without a total calorie surplus in your diet.

Now, there are many health and hormonal consequences that excess sugar can cause, and there are many different types of sugary food. More natural sugar, like the 20 grams of natural sugar that would be consumed when you eat an apple, will have a much different impact on your body and health than 20 grams of sugar from a candy bar. Plus, if you have a specific health condition that makes it difficult to control your blood sugar levels (such as diabetes), then you must limit the number of refined sugars and carbohydrates in your diet, even if you are controlling your calories.

But for most people who are controlling calories and their weight, eating mostly whole protein and produce and staying active, eating some sugar in moderation will not negatively affect weight loss or health.

Here's another sugar shocker ... I've been around the fitness industry for over 20 years and have attended many events, seminars and conferences, meeting many famous fitness and nutrition gurus for breakfast, lunch and dinner. You know that super lean fitness model, athlete or celebrity whose body you admire so much? They indulge in some sweet treats on occasion, a lot more than you may think! This news just doesn't make it into their social media, highlight reel.

At the end of the day, a successful diet (for health and weight loss) comes down to finding a way of eating that you will follow over the long haul, one that controls total calories, so you can achieve and maintain your best body composition and health. You should make sure the calories you eat are balanced in whatever way gets you to your best body while maintaining maximum energy and getting plenty of essential vitamins, minerals and macronutrients (protein, fat and yes, carbohydrates).

CHAPTER 15:
THE SCALE AND YOUR SANITY

From our earliest childhood visits to the doctor's waiting room, to daily visits to our bathroom, most of us have been conditioned to think that stepping on a scale to measure our body weight is the gold standard of measuring our health—and for far too many, our happiness. The use of a scale might have been more acceptable 50 years ago because of lesser medical knowledge because anyone could step on this cheap and non-invasive tool and get an answer and metric on their health in seconds.

Fortunately, we have better measuring and monitoring tools available now and know much more about metabolic science today; but unfortunately, this tool still lingers and people overly rely on it as 'judge and jury' of tracking their progress. Often it is regarded as a way to measure self-worth.

As a fitness professional, it's the most frustrating thing I encounter, as the scale is the most fearful assessment tool people battle with when they start a journey to improve their health and fitness.

So why even use it? Well, it's easy to say scrap the scale, but again I don't believe in 'all or nothing' and I don't think it's necessary to do that, as that would be like throwing the baby out with the bath water (as they say). The scale can help monitor your progress, and, from a physical perspective, it matters more as a monitoring tool for some people than others (especially if you are clinically obese or really overweight). But it's just one small assessment tool of many, and it can help or hinder your motivation and mindset if it's not understood correctly.

Far too many people let the number on a scale determine their happiness about their health and that itself is not healthy. People get down when the scale is up, and they get up when the scale is down. Don't do this!

Don't put all your trust and emotions into the number on a scale; it just measures your current bodyweight at a given time of the day and on that given day so many other fluctuating factors can determine your weight that you can continually be led down a path of endless frustration.

Giving too much attention to the scale is like listening to a pathological liar. You can ask it the same question many times a day and get a different answer every time. But if you don't look for more information beyond that number you will accept what it says as the final verdict of your progress, conditioning yourself to think a lower number is good and a higher number is bad. This can send you into a tailspin of emotional torture, which can sabotage your energy and efforts.

Remember, your bodyweight is just a small piece of information. It's one number, one data point. If your goal is to lose weight, you probably specifically want to lose fat and look leaner, right? Our bodies and our fat is what others see, and—let's admit it—that's what matters most to us.

Nobody needs to know what a scale shows when we step on it. What we look like and what we weigh are different things; there are many 'skinny-fat' people walking around with small bone structures but little muscle holding up those bones, poor health and fitness and a high body fat percentage for their size—but have a low bodyweight.

Your height is also a big determinant of bodyweight. In general, the taller you are the more weight you can carry on your bone structure. For many tall people, having a lower bodyweight than the average is far from an indication of health and wellness. It might actually be a red flag for some serious health issues, mentally and physically.

Muscle and bone are denser than fat. One pound of body fat takes up almost twice as much space as one pound of muscle. Stronger people with more muscle or larger structures often weigh more than weaker, smaller people. Stronger people aren't worse off because they're heavier; they're better off because they are strong and strength is connected to longevity.

Example:

Two people might both weigh 180 pounds. One has 15 percent body fat while the other has 28 percent body fat. The first person will be lean and muscular while the second will be softer and more at risk of a variety of health problems (because of the higher body fat percentage). But the scale doesn't know or tell you the difference. Body weight is not the same as body fat percentage.

Although the terms weight loss and fat loss get tossed into the same pot, they have many factors that make them different.

The first thing you should ask yourself when you want to desperately achieve a specific bodyweight is a simple, but powerful one-word, three-letter question: Why? Why is that number, that amount of weight you want the scale to show, important to you? Dig deep into the meaning behind it. Where did you come up with that number?

Scale weight changes constantly throughout the day. Any figure the scale reports to you is merely a snapshot of a moment in time. The number doesn't take a whole lot of time to change, or need a reason to shift. You can gain or lose two to three pounds in an hour without any apparent cause at all.

To prove this point about how fast and dramatic body weight changes can be, it is well known that athletes like boxers, UFC fighters and wrestlers can drastically move up and down weight classes before an event by changing their body weight. Some can change their weight by up to 30 pounds in just a couple days using extreme eating and exercising tactics. But the change to their weight is not a change in their body fat. Remember that the next time you are up five pounds in 24 hours and start to panic.

These changes on the scale occur mainly because scale weight is subject to the fluctuations of water. Your intake of water, or output of it as sweat, can cause your total body weight to shift up or down several pounds within any given day.

Water and salt balance in the body can cause seasonal shifts in your weight, too. When the weather heats up in the spring and summer season, your body uses a hormone called aldosterone to help you retain more fluid. So what looks like a summertime slip-up in your progress might just be your body's natural reaction to the warmer weather.

Lastly, your body has an adaptation process to hold onto things it is not getting enough of, which includes water. If you're not drinking enough water, your body will hold on to more of it (water retention), giving you that heavy bloated look and making you feel heavier, as it blurs your body's shape and normal muscle definition.

As a former competitive bodybuilder, I know what a drastic difference manipulating fluids in your body can make on the scale, not just when you're trying to go up and down to get into different weight classes but also how different it can make you look. Many bodybuilding contests have been won or lost solely on changes in water retention to achieve the 'dry' look. The first time my father saw me in contest shape, sporting the dry look, he said, "you look like a skinned rabbit!"

FUNNY BUNNY FOOD FACT:

"Did you know that rabbit meat, being almost pure protein, is so lean and low in fat that if you were stuck in the wilderness and all you had to eat was rabbit, you could still starve to death? Known as 'rabbit starvation' or 'protein poisoning' it was noted by many explorers and travelers, who relied on hunting local game for food. The lack of fat in the rabbit meat contributed to malnutrition and starvation. But hopefully you don't ever have to worry about that."

Back to your weight and water: make sure you give your body a consistent intake of water so it realizes it doesn't need to hold on to extra water and you will release water weight naturally.

Get this: Stressing over your scale weight, can make it go up! Numerous studies show a relationship between elevated cortisol levels (stress hormones) and higher weights. A five-year study of more than 5,000 people in Australia found that those who felt the most stress also gained the most weight during that time span.

Even worse, cortisol production due to stress has been linked to higher levels of abdominal fat in both women and men. Due to your body's hormonal signals, when you are stressed, your body doesn't know or care why; it just cares about your survival, so it fights to keep body fat packed around your organs for protection and in case of famine, leaving you with excess belly fat.

Stress is also one of the main triggers of over-eating or, as it is commonly known, emotional eating. Combine emotional eating with stressing and obsessing over the scale and you have a vicious cycle of heavier versus happier: Stress makes you eat. Over-eating and stressing increases your weight. Your weight makes you stress and you eat more ... and the cycle continues.

Bathroom visits also affect the weight on the bathroom scale. Motility is the polite way of saying 'how frequently you poop' which has a part to play in what your body weight can be. This rate varies from person to person. Your regularity can change based on what, and how often, you eat. (People with an extremely slow rate are said to have gastroparesis, or delayed gastric emptying). How much you chew your food, whether or not you drink water with meals, and how much you move can also influence your motility and body weight.

But wait, there's more to hammer down the point I'm making about the scale.

Do you travel a lot? Scale weight can be as erratic and prone to change as a flight schedule. High altitude air travel or visiting higher altitude areas can impact your weight by disrupting your body's water balance. Again, back to the example of the lean, mean pre-contest bodybuilders; many contestants will avoid flying too close to a contest date because of how it can mess up their water retention and leave them looking temporarily soft and not as shredded as they truly are. Travelling through many time zones and resultant jet lag also affects circadian rhythms, along with motility and even the bacteria in the gut microbiome.

LET'S GET REAL

Sometimes as people get older they set body weight goals that aren't at all based on their current reality. For example, they might set a goal to lose weight in an attempt to reach their college weight or their pre-children weight. But your body has put on muscle as well as fat since those days. It's possible that the only way to reach such a body weight would be to sacrifice lean muscle, health and happiness—and that's not what you want.

To hit a specific lower body weight just because that was what you weighed when you were younger could leave you feeling awful, weaker, or not even liking the way you look at that weight. Plus the life sacrifices you would probably have to make to achieve it, while balancing life demands like family, career and an aging body, is usually not worth the sacrifice.

The bottom line is that there's a big problem with thinking that hitting a certain number on a scale will make you happy. It won't.

It's more important to focus on how you feel, how your clothes fit, your body fat percentage and measurements, such as chest, arms, waist, hips, and thighs as well as blood markers. Don't forget to be kind to yourself and look after your mental health as well because you want to be around for as long as you can to enjoy your fitter body.

At my fitness facility, we have four steps we follow to assess and monitor our clients' body composition using the same tools under the same conditions each time.

1. Posture Progress Pictures: We take a photo of you simply standing relaxed with arms down by your side against a plain white backdrop with good lighting and minimal clothing. Photos are taken of front, each side and back. We then do two upper body mobility tests, "The Pen Test" and "The Behind the Back Scratch Test" to assess shoulder and upper back thoracic spine mobility and flexibility. I don't like to retake the photos any sooner than four weeks apart. But with consistent easy eating and exercise over many months you will notice the changes, not just in your progress, but in your posture as well.

2. Body Weight: Yes, I believe you should still use a scale to track your body weight, because the more information you have about the state of your body, the better, as indicators will change at different times. But remember, body weight is just one piece of data; it's not the be-all, end-all, because weight is just one measure of progress and success. Most importantly, do not check it every day. Once a week at most is enough.

3. Bodyfat Percentage: No, you don't have to get a personal trainer to pinch you with body fat-tracking calipers. Besides being uncomfortable, calipers are only as accurate as the pincher's touch with can cause huge variances in readings. If you have access to high-end diagnostics under the guidance of a professional (like a Dexa scanner, bod pod machine or underwater hydrostatic weighing), these are the most accurate ways to measure body fat.

But most of us don't have million-dollar contracts that depend on how we look or our exact body fat percentage, so try instead a simple handheld Omron Bodyfat Monitor (which we use at my fitness facility) which uses bio impedance to monitor body fat. This machine will provide consistent readings over time that are quite accurate. However, depending on your hydration, you can get fluctuations in this reading, so be consistent with your conditions when you use it and assess a trend over weeks and months, not days.

Bodysite Measurements: Get a soft body tape measure (several options like the MyoTape are available on Amazon) and measure yourself. I like to use five sites with my clients: mid-chest, mid-upper arm, waist around the belly button, hips around the widest part and across your backside, and mid-upper thigh. You can even measure small sites if you wish, like neck and calves. I like to just measure one side of the body as we have variances in the natural girth of our muscles from one side of our body to other.

Health and Happiness Markers: Make sure you get at least one annual medical examination to assess your basic health markers as well as the harder-to-quantify aspects of your health and wellness, like how you feel mentally and physically. Your energy, mood, how your clothes fit, as well as physical progressions in exercise performance are all markers of health and happiness.

The Final Weigh-in on Your Weight

Stop torturing yourself about your weight, because no one is judging you as hard as you are. No one really cares about that number. Seriously. Sharing our weight numbers has always been so taboo. We don't like to talk about it or even see the number when we step on the scale. I see so many clients who shield it likes it's their bank account number when writing it on their initial registration forms, or many just leave it out. In my office during a body composition assessment, many people step on the scale, close their eyes and cringe like they are standing on the edge of a cliff!

Think about this. When you begin to change your body and someone tells you that you look great, or even asks you if you lost weight, does the actual body weight number matter to you or them? It shouldn't. Remember, people only judge us physically at first glance. Once we know someone, they just look like themselves and we don't assess what their weight might be every time we see them. In the end, it's how we judge ourselves and how we feel about ourselves that matters most.

We constantly see having 'perfect' bodies in the media, from celebrities and athletes, to social media fitness freaks we are fed a false ideal of what is normal. First of all, like we used to say 20 years ago, "don't believe everything you see on T.V." Today that is expanded to, "don't believe everything you see and read on the internet." Would you change your opinion of these people if you found out they weighed ten more pounds than what you deemed ideal? No, because we judge by what we see, not by some arbitrary number.

We need to stop acting like our bodyweight is tattooed on our foreheads or printed on our shirts for the world to see! Imagine the freedom you would feel if you had no idea how much you weighed. So again. Repeat it with me: No one really cares.

CHAPTER 16:
THE MYTH OF MOTIVATION

It is four in the morning on a cold, rainy Monday as I write this, and I didn't necessarily feel motivated to get up and write this book before I get the kids off to school and go to work at the fitness facility that I run. But I have decided to pursue a life-long goal of writing this book and that requires making it a daily habit to sit down and write every day. For me, like many authors, it's easiest to write first thing in the early morning before my wife and two young kids wake up and the demands of the day start. Of course I'd rather be sleeping, doing it later, reading, making pizza—just about anything else—but instead I sit here bleeding words from my brain onto a screen and hoping this book eventually gets published so it helps people live healthier and happier lives.

Later today, after a busy morning coaching group workouts and operating my business, I will have to find the energy to squeeze in my *own* workout before I head out to pick up the kids from school and daycare. And even though fitness is what I love to do most, and the industry in which I have chosen to serve, many days I am not motivated to work out after giving so much of my mental and physical energy to training others and running my business.

If there is one main reason people come to me for fitness coaching, it's because they say they are not motivated to exercise or eat well on their own. Although I understand and believe in the role of a coach and a support system, it's the mindset around motivation that first needs to be trained.

Very often, we are filled with resistance when it comes to doing the things we want to do in our lives; don't let this resistance become an excuse not to do those things that you need and want to do.

I discovered a long time ago that motivation is overrated and believing it to be more important than it is can, ironically, be the thing that keeps us from reaching goals. That's right. Believing in the myth of motivation will derail you.

The common myth people generally fall for is the idea that you will only eat better, exercise and reach goals if you find the motivation to do so. The idea here is that magical motivation will grip you one day and it will be bigger and stronger than whatever resistance your brain and body can come up with.

But, resistance doesn't have to stop us, laziness doesn't have to stop us, discomfort, inconvenience, fear, exhaustion, weakness, even sickness doesn't have to stop us. You don't need to be motivated to do things. You just have to find a strong enough WHY and decide to act.

When clients say they want to achieve a goal but they are afraid, tired, inconvenienced or whatever, my answer is always, "That's okay. That's fine, that's normal, but you do what's important to you anyway."

You can dislike going to the gym and still make it there every day. You can feel lazy yet still take the steps necessary to start a business or write that book you always wanted to write. If you are waiting to be motivated, fearless, energetic or inspired, then you are setting yourself up for failure. You can keep your excuses; but don't let them stop you.

Yes, I know cake tastes better than salad. Hitting the snooze button is easier than getting up on a dark, depressing morning to go to work. And you probably would rather sit at home and watch Netflix than hit the gym. So would I, but I decided many years ago that my health, strength and energy are more import-ant than my need for motivation. And so there is no choice if you want to achieve health and fitness goals. Make it a habit, whether you feel like it or not. After 25 years of practicing these habits I don't even need to think about them. That's the secret: once you discover that your goals are more important than motivation, you will find ways to work to accomplish them.

Do you want to get something done? The good news is you don't really need motivation at all. You just need to take action, sooner rather than later. Any action is better than no action. You can always correct course and adjust along the way.

Newtons First Law: "The law of inertia. An object at rest stays at rest and an object in motion stays in motion."

If you want to get things done and reach goals, the number one predictor of success will simply be taking action. Are you ready to take action? If the answer is a resounding, "YES!" then let's get moving. Don't even think about it, just decide.

Here's how ...

Use this great strategy from motivational speaker and best-sell-ing author, Mel Robbins, who wrote the book, *The 5 Second Rule*.

The 5 Second Rule is simple. *"If you have an instinct to act on a goal, you must physically move within 5 seconds or your brain will kill it."*

Think about a new habit, like trying to get up earlier (and not hitting the snooze button) so you can get to the gym.

Those few seconds when you open your groggy eyes and you have that angel and devil dancing on your shoulder telling you to either get up or go back to sleep, are when you have to act. The minute you let thought and doubt (the devil) take over is the minute you lose and hit snooze. This is when you apply the 5 Second Rule. It's like ripping off a Band-Aid, it's fast and effective.

When you feel yourself hesitate before doing something that you know you should do, count down 5-4-3-2-1-GO and physically move towards action.

Physical movement and action are key to getting things done. They change your state of mind and break the 'habit loop' trap that is so easy to fall in to. And by counting backwards instead of falling back to sleep you are actually using neuroscience to change your thought patterns, habit-based loops controlled by your subconscious (based in the basal ganglia in the back part of your brain). The conscious, or the action-based, part of your brain is in the front (pre-frontal cortex) and is responsible for decision-making, planning and working towards goals. Counting down from five sounds silly I know, (I thought so too at first), but it is actually a powerful form of metacognition or the awareness and understanding of one's own thought processes, and is something anyone can do, anytime. It works.

There is a window that exists between the moment you have an instinct to change and the moment your mind talks you out of it. It's a five-second window. And it exists for everyone. If you do not take action on your instinct to change, you will stay stagnant. You will not change. But if you do that one simple thing, you can prevent your mind from working against you. You can start the momentum of change before the barrage of thoughts and excuses hit you with full force.

This is how you push yourself to do the hard stuff such as work you don't feel like doing, you're scared of, or you're avoiding. That's it. Five seconds is all it takes. If you don't act on an instinct within that five-second window, that's it. You won't be doing it.

David T. Neal, Wendy Wood, and Jeffrey M. Quinn in a 2002 to 2005 Duke university study showed at least 45 percent of our waking behavior is habitual. That's means almost half your daily actions are on automatic!

CHAPTER 17:
5 STEPS TO BUILDING A HEALTHY HABIT

1. Real Reason

Most people need to dig deep to find their 'why' behind their desire to change. Asking why you want to change something at least five times will get you to your most meaningful answer. Those who are most successful at adopting lifestyle changes usually find a 'why' that involves others, not themselves. Looking good at your friend's wedding not deep enough; being healthy and fit enough to walk your child down the aisle or play with your grandkids goes deeper.

2. Tripwire Trigger.

Most of the food or fitness related decisions we make are not only automatic but dictated by ones we made beforehand. Like stepping through a trip wire, we set traps for ourselves that activate events that blow up in our face later.

Do you cave in to salty and sweet carbohydrate cravings at night? That's because you probably skipped breakfast, didn't eat enough protein throughout the day or simply didn't get enough sleep. Not getting enough sleep can lead you to hitting the snooze button and blowing off your planned morning workout. That makes you wake up feeling sluggish mentally and physically ... and so you keep repeating the cycle of poor decisions. Address the cause, not the symptom.

3. Simple Swap.

I see this all the time in the dieting world. Someone decides to follow a low-carbohydrate diet and ditch the breads and grains on their plate. With the drastic drop in calories, of course they lose weight fast at first (mostly water weight from depleted muscle glycogen). But after a few weeks, because they dropped calories too drastically and didn't replace their starchy carbohydrates with more nutrient-dense (but lower calorie) fruits and vegetables, they cave in to chronic hunger and binge themselves back to square one. It's important to replace a bad habit or a poor food choice with something else more obviously beneficial to your goals. Choosing a flavored sparkling water instead of your normal wine or beer is just one example of a swap towards success.

4. Easy Eating and Exercise.

Build small wins at first when you're trying to change a health habit. It's important to choose something so small and easy that you think, "this is too easy! It's not going to make a difference!" Trust me, it will—if you practice your new habit. You need to ingrain easy habits *first* before you make them harder. The practice is actually more important than the habit at first.

Don't cook much at home? Cook just one healthy meal this weekend. I know what you are thinking. "That's too easy." Great! Easy to say or easy to do? Just do it first for two weeks before you say it's easy and once it actually becomes easy, then start cooking one healthy meal on a weekday, then eventually every single day if you can.

Not doing consistent exercise because you say you are too busy? Everyone has four minutes! Do one four-minute Tabata workout of squats and pushups using the Tabata protocol, which is 20 seconds of work and 10 seconds of rest, repeated for 8 rounds totalling 4 minutes. Perform squats for 20 seconds, then use the 10 seconds rest as transition time (to get in a pushup position on the floor), then perform pushups for 20 seconds. Repeat alternating those two exercises for eight total rounds for a four-minute total body workout that will challenge your muscles and metabolism. You can do this pretty much anywhere and at any time. Add additional days or four-minute rounds using new exercises to build up endurance and energy. Like achieving colored belts in martial arts, you need to practice exercise and eating until it's easy, then prove that you have earned the right to take on a greater challenge.

5. Prepare to Plan.

If your goals are important to you, you will find a way to achieve them. If they are not, you will find an excuse not to. Even after finding your important 'why,' identifying your triggers, making swaps from poor nutrient food to better stuff and practicing new habits until easy, you will still need to prioritize and plan how to fit it all together within the context of your busy life.

You will need to plug into what matters and schedule time in advance for the things that matter. Work time, family time, meal time and health and self-time. Monday to Sunday schedules need to be thought out ahead of time to the best of your abilities. We don't live in a bubble, so unexpected things will come up and that's normal. Be flexible and adaptable when they do but don't cheat yourself; get done what you planned. Planning and structure give you freedom—not the other way around, as many think. Be proactive with planning to build rock solid healthy habits.

> "If you really want to do something, you'll find a way. If you don't, you'll find an excuse."
>
> — Jim Rohn, Best Selling Author, Motivational Speaker

CHAPTER 18:
RECHARGE YOUR MIND, MUSCLES AND METABOLISM

THE SIMPLE SEVEN SLEEP SOLUTION

In order to get up earlier in the morning you need to get a good night's sleep, so that's where my Simple Seven Sleep Solution comes in.

Samuel L. Jackson said it so well in his famous voice-over of the children's book written by Adam Mansbach, "Go the F*** to Sleep!" But sleep isn't just for babies. It's for busy bodies like yours and mine.

It's not cool or healthy to be proud of running on fumes, or on only a few hours' sleep per night. Sure, we all have to do that at times, especially if you have young kids or are running your own business like me. But any successful person in their right mind who understands what is required to obtain health and happiness will tell you, we all need to get consistent, good quality sleep.

Loyola University Chicago Stritch School of Medicine researcher Lydia DonCarlos, PhD, is a member of an expert panel of 12 representatives, including Dr. DonCarlos, who were selected by medical organizations; and six sleep experts selected by the National Sleep Foundation that's making new recommendations on how much sleep people need. The panel, convened by the

National Sleep Foundation, is making its recommendations based on age, ranging from newborns (who need 14 to 17 hours of sleep per day) to adults aged 65 and up (7 to 8 hours per day).

These are the sleep-time recommendations from the National Sleep Foundation expert panel:

- Newborns (0-3 months): Sleep range narrowed to 14-17 hours each day (previously it was 12-18).

- Infants (4-11 months): Sleep range widened two hours to 12-15 hours (previously it was 14-15).

- Toddlers (1-2 years): Sleep range widened by one hour to 11-14 hours (previously it was 12-14).

- Preschoolers (3-5): Sleep range widened by one hour to 10-13 hours (previously it was 11-13).

- School age children (6-13): Sleep range widened by one hour to 9-11 hours (previously it was 10-11).

- Teenagers (14-17): Sleep range widened by one hour to 8-10 hours (previously it was 8.5-9.5).

- Younger adults (18-25): Sleep range is 7-9 hours (new age category).

- Adults (26-64): Sleep range did not change and remains 7-9 hours.

- Older adults (65+): Sleep range is 7-8 hours (new age category).

However, sleep quality matters just as much as quantity. (Seven hours is the magic number that keeps me charged up; any less than six hours comes back to haunt me after a few days). Research also shows that getting less than six hours' sleep per night for five consecutive nights puts your body's insulin sensitivity close to diabetic levels!

But if you're not getting enough sleep, keep the sleep medication behind the counter and off your night table and use my **Simple Seven Sleep Solution** to help you wind down naturally at night instead.

#1. Set a wake time but also a bed time at least **SEVEN** hours before you want to get up and stick to it as best you can. Even set a reminder alarm for 15 to 30 minutes before bed to remind you to get ready for bed, then shut down your day and go to bed. As a driven entrepreneur and busy parent, I get up extremely early (4:00 a.m.), so I have to bite the bullet and be in bed by 8:30 p.m. and asleep by 9:00 p.m. at the latest.

#2. SEVEN hours before your scheduled bed time, stop consuming caffeine. Caffeine packs a powerful punch and is great to crank you up early in the day—and coffee has proven health and fat loss benefits—but caffeine has a half-life in your system for six to eight hours for most people and can greatly interfere with winding you down. I cut the caffeine by 1p.m., giving me an eight-hour opportunity to wind down before I sleep so I am not staring at the ceiling, wired and not tired, at bedtime. As for alcohol, it helps relax you initially, and even doze off, but it actually worsens your quality of sleep in the long run so don't use it as a nightcap.

#3. Eliminate most electronics from your room (like TV and phone) and read a real paper book or even the new Amazon Kindle Paperwhite (it doesn't use bright blue light to keep your brain lit up). Then flood your monkey mind with feel-good thoughts by writing in a Gratitude Journal, noting **SEVEN** things you are grateful for or that you accomplished that day; big or small, everything counts. If you fall asleep before getting to seven, the plan worked perfectly, so be grateful.

These tips will give your busy body and brain the best environment for a good night's sleep without having to battle any effects from something in a bottle. Sweet dreams!

CHAPTER 19:
TURN GOAL SETTING INTO GOAL GETTING

Sounds too simple, but writing a few sentences down and having them visible where you can see them often can mean the difference between success and failure. Plenty of studies show that people who write their goals down on paper and consistently see them are five to ten times as likely to achieve them.

FOCUS ON YOUR BEHAVIOR BASED GOALS NOT YOUR OUTCOME BASED GOALS

But even when people do write out their goals, many focus on the outcome (like losing 20 pounds) instead of the behavior changes they should be focusing on to get there. You never have direct control of outcomes, despite your best efforts. Outcomes are affected by external stressors such as your crazy busy job, your sick child or parent, the gym being closed, exams to study for, bills to pay. You know; real life! Habits are not. Habits can be derailed for an hour or a day, but they remain habits.

Other things that can affect us are internal physical things we have little control over, such as hormone fluctuations (which affect energy and metabolism), chronic injury, a tough flu or a chronic disease. Here are some others: poor sleep. Travelling. Back pain. Knee pain. Shoulder pain. Just the pain of getting older.

You get the idea. You can't make your body do exactly what you want it to (and neither can your personal trainer), but you do have control of your daily efforts or your 'behavior-based' goals, like 'exercise today for 30 minutes,' or, 'eat a healthy salad for lunch.'

SMALL HINGES SWING BIG DOORS

Just as we want to make eating easy, let's make 'goal setting and goal getting' not just easier but more effective by focusing on our daily behaviors combined with the proven and practical S.M.A.R.T Start System.

A goal must be **Specific, Measurable, Attainable, Realistic and Timely.**

A good goal is specific enough to direct your focus on the change that's most needed or important to you. 'I will get fit this year' doesn't really give you anything measurable or specific to work on.

However, 'I will lose five percent of my body fat,' does. It's specific to one area of improvement and measurement (body fat) and it includes a measurable outcome (five percent).

Goals should be challenging but realistic. They must be big enough to inspire you to action with some sense of urgency and accountability, but not so big that you get frustrated with the impossibility of accomplishing them.

If you're 50 pounds overweight, setting a goal of having a ripped six-pack of abdominal muscles in three months isn't realistic for most people.

On the other hand, setting a goal to lose ten pounds over the next twelve months, while realistic, lacks enough urgency and is just too small for most to be inspiring.

Many people don't realize what good progress is and expect results yesterday. For weight loss, losing one-half to one pound of body weight per week on average is actually great progress! Most people don't jump for joy if they lose four pounds in a month because it seems so slow they're not even sure if it happened. You can lose that much body weight in a week—or even a couple days—but it will just be water weight, not body fat. But by doing it right, losing an average of four pounds a month over just three months can have your weight down twelve pounds!

If you have more weight to lose, just add more months, as the progress will slow down as you lose more weight. Don't expect to lose weight as fast in month six as you did in week six. Change your expectations. Losing one-quarter to one-half a pound a week on average is still considered good progress, bringing you down three to six pounds in three months. Doesn't sound like much right? But hold three to six sticks of butter in your hand and tell me you wouldn't be happy losing that much off your body? Remember, the faster you lose the weight the harder it's going to be to maintain the weight loss.

If you have to turn your life upside down to get your weight to go down, eventually you will go back to your old habits and your body will fight to bring your weight back up. So give yourself some time to get to your best body and then settle in to maintain it. Some studies show it can take as long as 18 months for your body to get comfortable with your new body composition numbers.

Once your goals are written down, share them; don't keep them a secret! If a goal is a secret, it's easy to blow it off when things get tough. The real secret to staying consistent and achieving goals is accountability. If you've got at least one person or, even better, a group of supportive people holding you accountable to your new behavior, you're way more likely to succeed. That's why the group fitness training and one-on-one nutrition consulting we offer at my fitness business work so well.

So build a 'best team' around you by using the positive power of a good coach, supportive friends and an online community.

> "Focus on your behavior based goals, not your outcome based goals."
>
> — Dr. John Berardi, Precision Nutrition

CHAPTER 20:
THE BIGGEST MINDSET MISTAKE

WHY YOU KEEP STARTING AND STOPPING

"I'll get back to healthy eating and exercising after my vacation ... once the kids go back to school in September ... after Dad gets out of the hospital ... In the New Year ..."

While this kind of 'all or nothing' or 'on and off mentality' is all too common, it leads to pausing, not progress, and usually nothing gets achieved in terms of sustainable results. Why? Because it doesn't teach you how to balance exercise and eating well within the demands of real life.

There is no perfect time to get fit and lose weight and if you start and stop every time life's challenges come up, you will never get anywhere. If there is any secret at all to making healthy habits stick as a lifestyle it's having the ability to be flexible and pivot around real life demands, not giving up the minute you miss your scheduled workout or forget your healthy, packed lunch at home.

> "The tree that does not bend with the wind will be broken by the wind."
>
> *— Chinese proverb*

Your health and fitness can't be played like a movie where you simply hit 'pause' or 'play' when something comes up to distract you. Life, and making progress toward anything, doesn't work that way. You need to expect things to come up, because they will. The most successful people anticipate and plan for challenges; they are not reactive, they are responsive and they don't crumble when obstacles arise.

So, just like in life, which also has no pause button, the idea is to practice doing your best with your healthy habits during all of life's circumstances. That's why people who succeed in changing their bodies learn to adapt and dial up or down their efforts as needed.

I like to use the analogy of a flame on a propane burner. The secret of success is to dial the flame up or down when needed but never to shut it off. Any positive effort, no matter how small, is better than totally giving up. Maintaining even a small pilot light on a burner is better than having no flame at all and it makes it easier to dial it back up when the time is right.

Change is hard, especially at first. But the more you realize that sometimes 30 percent change is better than zero percent, the better and easier it will get. I believe this 'pause button mentality' only builds the habit of pausing and encourages people to constantly chase perfection, instead of steadily making progress. Always be something—not all or nothing.

> "Don't be all or nothing, be always something."
>
> — Dr. Krista Dixon Scott, Precision Nutrition

CHAPTER 21:
COMPLIANCE CALENDAR.

DON'T BREAK THE CHAIN

You've probably heard it takes 21 days to develop a habit, but the real research shows it actually takes at least 66 days and often longer. This is one of the most important things I've learned. Other good advice I received about habit-building and achieving success was from the successful comedian Jerry Seinfeld.

Asked by a young aspiring comedian how he got so good and how he comes up with new material, he said, "write something every day and don't break the chain." Jerry would make it a goal and game to write jokes every single day and when he did he marked an "X" on his calendar. The goal was to not break the chain of Xs, allowing him to see the consistency of sticking to habits that ultimately made him successful. I think it worked, don't you?

This technique can work for any healthy habit you want to make stick. I use a 'Compliance Calendar' and it has worked tremendously for me and many of my clients. Pick one, or two at most, new habits to work on for the next 66 days, get a calendar out and post it where you will see it. Even better, post it where others will see it too, to hold you accountable.

For example, pick one habit for better eating, another for more exercise. Each day you complete your goal of better eating (like eating protein and produce meals three times a day) mark one stroke of the X from corner to corner on the date box.

If you complete your daily exercise habit, (like a 30-minute workout) mark a stroke in the other direction on the date, completing the X.

For the next 66 days, try not to break the chain of Xs. Do you need to be perfect to see results? Absolutely not. You just need to focus on progress and go for the longest streaks you can on the compliance calendar. If at the end of 66 days you have at least 50 days of Xs you will have achieved around 80 percent compliance, which is where most of us need to be to make good progress. Let the other 20 percent be for life's indulgences, pure experience and enjoyment. Whatever your score, always try to beat and better it. Be unbreakable and don't break the chain. "That's gold Jerry, gold!" - Kenny Bania, Seinfield

CHAPTER 22:
THE DIRTY DIET

Eating clean: it's a common label used in the fitness and nutrition world for eating healthy. But what is the line we are drawing in the dirt to decide what eating clean really is?

I think the concept of eating clean is one way we make something essential, like eating, too rigid and complicated, causing more stress and unnecessary food guilt that many times is worse than the food itself.

Whether it's the 'clean fifteen' organic foods versus the 'dirty dozen, both shown below,' or local slow food versus filthy fast food, just sticking with real foods that come from a farm and not a factory most of the time will give you your best body without you having to obsess over calories or feel deprived.

The Dirty Dozen" list includes: celery, peaches, strawberries, apples, domestic blueberries, nectarines, sweet bell peppers, spinach, kale, collard greens, cherries, potatoes, imported grapes and lettuce.

"The Clean 15" bore little to no traces of pesticides, and is safe to consume in non-organic form.
This list includes: onions, avocados, sweet corn, pineapples, mango, sweet peas, asparagus, kiwi fruit, cabbage, eggplant, cantaloupe, watermelon, grapefruit, sweet potatoes, sweet onions

Personally I like to choose local and fresh over organic, as many local small farms grow and produce healthy, natural food. Getting organic certification is costly and time- intensive and is not feasible for many small producers. Plus here in Eastern Canada, I am not willing to pay double for organic produce that is half-rotten and leaves a huge environmental footprint to travel across the planet to get to my supermarket shelf.

But if some organics (usually within the 'dirty dozen') look fairly fresh and have a practical price, I will choose them when possible. In the end the most important thing is eating broccoli consistently, not whether or not broccoli is a superfood, certified organic and grown in a vacuum on the moon.

As for general health and body composition, a magical thing happens when you eat real food. You get the nutrients you need and you get filled up naturally when you should, which prevents overeating too many calories in the long term. Have you ever eaten a whole bag of apples? Probably not. How about a bag of chips? Probably. Even the most stringent of nutrition fanatics have probably found their way to the bottom of a chip bag.

But guess what? It's okay. Just follow the 80-20 rule, which means that 80 percent of the foods you eat determine your health and body shape, so stick with good nutritious real whole foods 80 percent of the time. Also be mindful and take the time to eat until you're also 80 percent satisfied, not stuffed like a pizza pocket.

The other 20 percent of the time enjoy an occasional pizza or pint with your friends. No stress, no guilt and no gut, when kept in proper balance.

One of the biggest benefits of exercising and consistently eating well is having extra wiggle room to enjoy the 'dirty' foods every now and again along with the people and experiences that come on the side. If you think back, some of your fondest memories probably revolve around food.

Sure, food is meant to nourish us, but it is also meant to be enjoyed. So enjoy your eating—clean and dirty—and keep it real 80 percent of the time. Remember, some of the cleanest foods come from the ground.

> "Food is meant to nourish us but it is also meant to be enjoyed."
>
> —Sean Barker

CHAPTER 23:
MINDLESS MONDAYS

You can do your food preparation whenever you want to, but many people like Sunday and Wednesday best. But be ready for the start of the week, or at least try to make Monday mindless. The point is to remove the friction of eating on the fly because you will make poor choices. Anticipate being busy during the work week and plan and pack meals ahead of time as much as you can.

Easy Eating Tip: Eat the exact same breakfast, lunch and dinner, at least every Monday. Avoid thinking to start the week, resist the urge to change the plan and relish the routine. Just eat the same things on Mondays or whatever day starts your working week. Then feel free to make the other days easy by using the additional Simple Swap options. Remember, let's make eating easy!

THE EASY EATING MINDLESS MONDAY MEAL PLAN

Breakfast

- **60 Second Simple Supershake**
- 1 scoop of whey or plant protein
- 1 banana
- Handful of pre-washed baby spinach
- Blend in water and ice, or use a frozen banana instead of fresh

- Fish Oil Omega 3 supplement: 4 capsules or 2 tsp of fruit flavoured liquid

Simple Swaps: instead of a shake, choose 1 serving of plain Greek yogurt or cottage cheese with berries, or breakfast meats or eggs/egg whites. (You need at least 20 to 30 grams of protein in the morning to feel satiated throughout the day, control blood sugar and enhance metabolism).

Instead of a banana, you can choose an apple or orange on the side, or berries blended or any serving of fruit. Kale or greens powder can be used to add good greens variety to a shake. Cooking in coconut oil, avocado oil, olive oil or butter can provide some fat, but nothing comes close to replacing fish oil for pure omega-3s (just don't cook with fish oil!).

Lunch

- **Grab and Go Finger Foods**
- Natural Nitrate Free Deli Turkey- 4 rolled slices
- 1 Apple
- 10 Almonds

Simple Swaps: instead of deli turkey, try any natural deli meats that you like rolled up, such as roast beef, ham, or chicken. Or swap the deli meat with any pre-cooked or prepared sliced meat protein from roasted chicken, beef, turkey, tuna or eggs. Swap the apple with another choice of fruit or even a mixed green salad. Swap the almonds with two thumb size servings of cubed cheese. Or if you didn't have a super shake for breakfast, you can have one for lunch. Halfway through the day and no cooking required; now that's easy eating!

Dinner

30-Minute Meal

- Lean Ground Beef- palm sized burger patty fried or grilled
- Small Baked Potato (poke with fork, wrap in paper towel and microwave for 5 minutes)
- Frozen Bag Broccoli Florets: 1 cup (microwave for 5-8 minutes in covered bowl or steam)
- 1 Tbsp of extra virgin olive oil on cooked broccoli and 1 tbsp of melted butter on potato or fat free sour cream
- Season with spices of choice, or a one and done garlic multi-spice blend for fast flavour!

Simple Swaps: instead of ground beef, try ground chicken, ground turkey, ground pork, ground sausage or any meat protein you desire in a simple recipe with some vegetables and a different controlled starchy carbohydrate portion like rice or pasta. A roasted deli chicken or beef roast, or fish fillets. Chili, soup, stew, stir-fry, a casserole or just protein, produce, starch foods paired on the plate.

*Adjust servings up or down depending on your weight, activity level and goals.

THE HOW AND WHY

The key in all of this is mindless eating to remove the decision fatigue, time and fuss so you can start your week with momentum. If you look at this Monday meal plan, you'll see everything is easy. Easy to buy, easy to prepare, easy to eat! Easy is good when you are looking for less friction and faster fat loss.

Start the day with a minute meal for breakfast, such as the Simple Super Shake. Eat a good source of protein to kick-start your day and enhance metabolism and muscle recovery. Add some ready, easy-to-use pre-washed spinach and you won't even taste it after it gets pulverized in the blender. This will give you some good greens. Add a banana for texture and essential energy and you're on easy eating street. Pop your fish oil capsules or throw fruit flavored fish oil in your shake if you use the liquid. Breakfast mastered in a minute. You're on with your day.

We all get busy at lunch, and many times we are away from home, so for no cooking required lunch, grab some natural deli turkey slices, or deli chicken or roast beef slices, or whole deli-roasted, ready-to-go BBQ chicken from the market—whatever you like for pre-cooked meat protein. Eat an apple and some almonds and your easy eating day is looking lean and healthy so far!

Dinner is the only meal that requires some actual cooking and is usually the one we like to sit down and take time to eat. I've made that easy for you. I am sure you can commit at least 30 minutes a day to eating healthy? Get a palm-size amount of ground beef, or ground turkey or chicken if you like. Cook it up in one tablespoon of oil either crumbled or as a burger patty; add some spice and a little side of starch (a small cooked potato is easily done in the microwave).

When the potato is done, cool it and toss frozen broccoli florets in a bowl to cook in the microwave. It doesn't have to be broccoli; Brussels sprouts, asparagus, green beans, cauliflower or mixed veggies are all fine. Just buy it in bulk and pack your freezer with it. Frozen vegetables are easy and just as nutritious as fresh. Besides microwaving, you can steam, sauté, or bake them in the oven with olive oil until golden brown. Whatever works!

Everything in this easy eating meal plan has been deliberately made as EASY as it can be, especially for when you start your work week. These meals don't take much time or thought and you only need to cook one meal a day—and even that you can prep days before if you wish.

If cooking for two or more people, multiply the servings as needed but control the servings on your own plate. You are doing this for *you*, and to change your body, so you have to be responsible for what goes into your mouth. Women should generally eat a palm size portion of protein, a fist-size portion of veggies, a cupped-hand size portion of starchy carbohydrates (around 1/2 a measured cup). Men (who are generally larger and have more muscle) can double those suggested servings.

Don't obsess about exactly measuring every ounce and calorie in your food! Eyeball it the best you can and use your weight loss tracker guide to determine if you need to eat less or more based on your weekly weight change. Once you control portions for a few weeks, weight loss will follow. You can also adjust to your satiety and activity level. Stop eating before you're stuffed and if you are highly active (five hours of activity a week) you can get away with eating a little more.

Like I mentioned in the simple swaps section of this book, feel free to try different proteins and produce throughout the week but only if it's easy for you to plan and prepare them. Substitute kale for spinach in your morning smoothie. Use leftover roasted chicken or sliced roast beef in your lunch. Eat an orange instead of an apple. Have rice or pasta instead of potatoes for dinner. But if you start getting fancier than that, you will likely go off track with your new habits. When in doubt, hit the easy eating button and follow the plan to the letter; at least for Monday stay within the guidelines.

Emergency Easy Eating Meal.

Life happens, so be flexible or 'be like water' as Bruce Lee said. I think he knew something about being fit and lean!

If you are out and about and get caught unprepared to eat according to your food plan, here's an easy option to replace a meal.

For breakfast, a small Egg McMuffin or an egg and veggie breakfast burrito at McDonalds, or similar fast food options, provide the lowest calories.

For lunch or dinner, any small half size Chicken or Cobb Salad at a fast-food restaurant is acceptable. Yes, ask for a small salad because, especially at some popular family restaurants, some salads can be 1,000 calories or more! Choose a balsamic vinegar-based dressing on the side. A chicken salad can be picked up at any drive-thru in any town. No excuses, easy-peasy.

> "When you strive for greatness, chaos is guaranteed to show up."
>
> *— Francis Ford Coppola,*
> *Famous American Movie Producer*

HOW MANY CALORIES?

This has to the number one question I get—how many calories should I eat? I know and have tons of formulas to use as a guide. But in most cases I don't. I am a real life test-and-adjust kind of coach. Everyone is different. I hate math, and you don't have to use a calculator to eat and lose fat.

I lost 30 pounds and got down to a ripped five percent body fat in 12 weeks for bodybuilding contests back in the day and technically I did not obsess and track every calorie. I was also runner-up in a world-wide body transformation contest and I used the same method, gradually eating a little less and exercising a little more. I have helped thousands of people achieve similar results, so

I know what works. I set a base calorie range for a high protein, moderate carbohydrate diet; followed it in week one; tweaked my meal plan based on bodily changes; dropped a little extra carbohydrates every two weeks; and, added a little extra exercise along the way depending on progress.

Set a consistent intake base first, see if your weight changes after a week or two and only after that test and tweak your plan based on your weight loss and how you feel. Let your personal progress and life be your ultimate fat loss guide. Keeping a food journal can keep you on target. At the end of the week, average your daily caloric intake to see how it compares to your weight.

AM I EATING THE RIGHT AMOUNT OF CALORIES?

If you lose more than three pounds a week consistently, you're not eating enough.

If you're losing one to two pounds per week, you're eating the right amount for fat loss.

If your weight is staying the same, you're eating appropriately for maintenance.

If you gain weight you're simply eating too many calories.

CHAPTER 24:
5 DRIVE-THRU HEALTHY HACKS FOR FITTER FAST FOOD

Picture this: Soccer and gymnastic practice ran late for the kiddos and you need to feed the family before they chew the leather off the seats of the car. They are fighting with you to pull over at their favorite drive-thru restaurant and fighting among themselves about which one to choose. You have been diligent about going to the gym and banishing your belly so you don't want to cave in and have a calorie bomb of cheeseburgers, fries and soda. Plus the sodium content alone will have your doctor literally twisting your arm to get better blood pressure results during your next medical.

But all is not lost if you use this Drive-Thru Healthy Hack guide to still get a fast food fix and feel good about the choices you make for you and your family.

When it comes to fast food, focus on the best choices instead of the perfect choices. Remember, perfect is the enemy of good at the drive-thru window—as well as at any of life's windows of opportunity.

#1. Go Grilled

Almost every fast food chain offers some form of grilled chicken salad or even grilled beef burgers instead of fried breaded chicken or saturated fat-soaked burger patties. Even if it's not really 'grilled,' choosing grilled or broiled meat will save you calories, sodium and fat. Watch out with salads, though. Sometimes the calories in the dressing are worse than those in the burgers, so ask for a balsamic vinegar-based dressing, or only use half of the cream-based dressing.

Do you really want a burger? Have one then, but choose the smallest one they offer, ask for no cheese and double the veggies, like lettuce, tomato and onion. Watch mayonnaise-based special sauces as they alone can add hundreds of calories in fat to a burger, so stick with mustard and a little ketchup and you'll be fine. If you do break down and get a bigger burger, make a happy deal with yourself and get a small side salad instead of fries.

#2. Choose Chili.

Chili is probably one of the best protein and fiber-packed choices you can make at many fast food chains. The beef will not be grass-fed, organic meat from the mountains of Peru and the beans might have you keeping your window down, but you could do a lot worse. Also, if they serve a baked potato that could make for some good post-workout carbohydrates, but stay away from the cheese sauce and sour cream which add hundreds of extra calories. Spice it up old school with pepper and chives.

#3. Lean Liquids

The simple switch of choosing water, white milk (not a milkshake) or even diet soda over regular soda or sweetened ice tea can save you 500 calories per meal. Smart drink choices also keep you from punching your pancreas with a handful of sugar and keeps you off the waiting list for diabetes or insulin resistance.

#4. Drive Past the Drive-Thru

Sometimes waiting in line at the drive-thru takes longer than walking in and ordering something at the counter; get out of your car. Or instead, choose a good local deli sandwich shop and opt for something like freshly-sliced turkey on a whole-grain bun with veggie toppings to keep the food real and the calories controlled. Fruit, side salads or soups usually are freshly made and available and they will give you more nutritional bang for your buck.

#5. If You Fail to Plan, You Plan to Fail

Before you leave the house to begin your daily job as the kids' chauffeur, make sure to have simple snacks and a small case of bottled water in your car. Protein bars, mixed nuts or beef jerky are great grab-and-go options that won't stink up your car and blow up your belly—and they will keep teeth marks off your seats as well.

With these fast food healthy hacks you won't fear the site of the drive-thru and you will be resourceful not remorseful.

CHAPTER 25:
40 SUCCESS SECRETS TO BE HEALTHIER AND HAPPIER

THE FIVE PILLARS OF PROGRESS

1. **Plan and Prepare**. Go through your week's commitments on Sunday and organize your time based on your priorities for family, fitness and finances.

2. **Count on a Coach**. Get a professional coach in the field you need help with the most to direct you forward faster and hold you accountable along the way.

3. **Social Support**.

Be part of a group of like-minded people who are positive and supportive of your goals and dreams. Even online support is better than none.

> *"You are the average of the five people you surround yourself with."*
>
> — Jim Rohn. Best selling author and motivational speaker

4. **Make it Meaningful**. Figure out what's truly important to you and find *your* big reason for why you are working towards the goals you are. Ask yourself 'why' five times to find your real reason.

5. **Deadlines not Dreams**. You must create specific deadlines to give you a sense of urgency and make every day count, or you will slack off or give up when things get challenging.

6. **Efficient Exercise**. Doing metabolic resistance training for 30-minutes, three to four days a week is best for most busy people for a maximum training effect in the minimum amount of time. MRT (Metabolic Resistance Training) builds lean muscle and strength and creates a heightened metabolic after-burn to burn fat and shape your body. On other days, try enjoyable and less intense activities like walking or short bodyweight workouts to get at least four hours of total activity a week.

7. **Protein and Produce**. Eat real, whole protein and produce at least 80 percent of the time such as lean meats, fruits and vegetables. The other 20 percent, stick with some starchy car-bohydrates, if appropriate for you, or add healthy fats to meet your energy demands and health goals. Enjoy a few favorite treats once a week.

8. **Sleep Soundly**. Your life and longevity depends on good quality sleep more than you think it does. Focus on quality over quantity but any less than seven hours a night of consistent sleep will not leave you functioning at your best. Have a wind-down ritual every night, don't use electronics an hour before bed and sleep in a cool dark room. Use ear plugs and a sleep mask if needed.

9. **Simple Supplements**. Supplement only with essential nutrients that you are not getting through eating whole foods. No synthetic supplement comes close to matching the nutrients in real food. But most of us could use some supplements in the form of extra

vitamins, minerals, essential fatty acids and protein to nourish our busy brains and bodies. Have a multivitamin, extra vitamin C, D, omega-3, a probiotic and magnesium—this should cover the basics of what most people need more of.

10. **Toss out Temptation**. Protect your eating environment at home by keeping only healthy foods in your house. Willpower is limited so don't depend on it. If a trigger food is in your house, it will get eaten, no matter what your intentions. So make healthy eating easy and unhealthy eating hard.

11. **Manage your Mess**. Stress *kills*. Chronic stress due to work, finances and family that's not managed will hold back even the most ambitious exercise and eating plans. Prioritize your time and schedule time to de-stress or it will catch up to you and knock you down. Use meditation, mindfulness and practice gratitude; these things are proven to work and have stood the test of time.

12. **Freedom Formula**. Structure = Discipline = Power. You never get a day back, so plan for it. Then stick to your plan as much as possible and get your life power back.

13. **Morning Magic**. Get up at least 15 minutes earlier than you normally do, grab a pen and paper, focus on the biggest priority or challenge in your life and plan and prepare for meeting it. There is something magical about the early morning hours when your body and brain have a clean slate with no distractions. You won't miss 15 minutes more sleep, but you *will* get ahead of the demands of the day and get back enough time to turn your problems into progress.

14. **Prioritize and Preview**. A perfect day starts the night before as you plan for the next day, anticipating obstacles so you can be prepared ahead of time. Also, a brain dump at the end of each work day (writing down all the things on your mind) helps clear

your head and leaves you with a written reference about what to tackle the next day.

15. **Progress not Perfection Prevents Procrastination**. Try saying that fast! There is never a perfect time to start anything. Just start, then correct course as you get moving. If you don't *do* anything, you don't *get* anything.

16. **Control, Conquer, Concentrate**. Only spend energy and effort on what you can control in life. Learn to cope with what you can't control and only concentrate on what counts.

17. **Be the Boss**. It's your life, so make it easier by setting some rules. What you eat, whom you associate with and how you spend your time are important to consider. With structure comes freedom.

18. **Pick your Passion**. Your passion or work will take up the biggest part of your life so try to find work you love. If you do, you will never 'work' a day in your life. Well actually you will work more, but you will at least enjoy it.

19. **Leave a Legacy**. Once you find your passion, do your best to make a positive impact with it so you can help others now and long after you are gone.

20. **Crush Criticism**. Don't let the opinions of others get you down or hold you back. Opinions are just opinions, based on someone's thoughts and beliefs and they don't define you. When you focus on your important targets and stick to your guns others won't be able to shoot you down.

21. **Be Proactive not Reactive**. Be the captain of your own ship and plan and anticipate obstacles ahead. Don't get caught in a wreck because you were reactive instead of proactive.

22. **Live to Learn**. Continue to learn and work on getting better in all aspects of your life. Continue to challenge yourself and get out of your comfort zone.

23. **Think like a Tank**. Whatever obstacles come your way in life, think like a tank. Meet them head-on, strong and unstoppable, and keep rolling forward no matter how slow you go. Crush anything in your path that tries to stop you, no matter how difficult the battle.

24. **Be Extraordinary at Everything**. The world does not reward average people. Be extraordinary in everything you do. How you do anything is how you do everything. There is no traffic on the extra mile.

25. **Everyday Excellence**. Get better every day. Wake up every day and strive to be better in at least one facet of your daily life. If you are not growing, you are dying.

26. **Face your Flaws**. Be open and vulnerable. That's the only way people will know, like and trust you. The perfection of being human is our imperfections.

27. **Manners Matter**. Be polite and courteous. Always say please and thank-you, no matter to who or how often. Hold open doors and treat waiters with respect.

28. **Patience and Persistence**. The best things come to those who take little actions over a long time. Slow and steady wins the race.

29. **Surround Yourself with Support**. Surround yourself with positive and supportive people. You are the average of the five people who you surround yourself with.

30. **Build your Bookshelf**. Read at least a new book a month and build some mental muscle while you learn life lessons. You never get dumber by reading a book.

31. **Live and Lead**. Live by example and be your 'big self' by leading on your path to make it easier for others along the way.

32. **Experiences over Expenses**. The people you meet and the experiences you have, matter more than money or things.

33. **Leave them Laughing**. Make time to laugh every day. Even better, make someone else laugh with you. Leave everyone better than when you found them.

34. **Believe don't Break**. Believe in the unbreakable power of the human spirit. As long as you have air in your lungs you can get through anything. Don't get too high when things are good, or too low when things seem bad.

35. **Life not Loss**. When suffering through the loss of a friend or family member, as hard as it is, celebrate the life they lived instead of mourning their loss. Give grief time, as time heals all wounds. Scars are stronger than skin and memories last forever.

36. **Relish your Reputation**. It takes years to build your reputation but it can fall apart in a day, so make sure it's built on a strong foundation.

37. **Myth of Motivation**. Don't wait for motivation to get moving; get moving first and motivation and momentum will come. Taking action alleviates anxiety, so anytime you start thinking and not doing, count 5-4-3-2-1 to break the brain loop and go!

38. **Don't Be All or Nothing, Always Be Something**. If you get a flat tire on your car, would you then slash the other three? I hope not. So don't give up on your goals when you have a bad day, or even a bad week. Get back on the road right away and do something positive to move yourself in the right direction. No matter how small, movement is better than moping.

39. **Attitude of Gratitude**. The happiest and most successful people in the world (not necessarily the richest), live with an

attitude of gratitude no matter how much or little they have. Remember, when times get tough, someone out there has it more rough. Writing down at least one thing you are grateful for every day gives perspective and peace.

40. **Never say Never**. Always do the best you can, with what you have, where you are, and you will live a healthier and happier life.

> "Do what you can, with what you have, where you are."
>
> —Theodore Roosevelt, 26th American President

CHAPTER 26:
SIMPLE SHAKER SALAD RECIPES

If you are like me, you probably have a busy lifestyle to keep up with which makes eating healthy, and especially eating lots of veggies, pretty challenging at times. We all know that a good, hearty salad is good for you; however, due to everyone's busy and demanding schedules, finding time to prepare a good salad isn't always practical.

You can get salads in many fast food restaurants; unfortunately, most fast food salads are either not fresh, contains processed fillers, or their dressing contains more calories than a hamburger.

What most people don't know is that many fast food restaurants actually spray their salads with a substance made of propylene glycol to make their lettuce and other vegetables appear fresh, when they might actually be up to five days old! But choosing a fast food salad is still better for your body than the burger and fries, though these things are not the definition of eating well.

But I am about to reveal an ingenious way to prepare a tasty and healthy salad in a mason jar that can last for up to seven days (without a chemical spray). The secret is knowing how to layer the ingredients properly.

Here's to a simple way to shake up your diet with these **Simple Shaker Salads** to go!

HERE ARE THE THREE LAYERS:

The bottom layer is your salad dressing.

The middle layer is your harder, dense ingredients (to separate your top and bottom ingredients). These include carrots, cucumbers, cherry tomatoes, mushrooms, broccoli, peas, orange slices, beans, grains, and bell peppers. Then add in cooked chicken, steak, bacon, or chopped high quality natural deli meats in the middle layer.

> **Hint**: Keep the harder ingredients at the bottom (i.e carrots) since they don't absorb as much liquid.

The top layer is your leafy vegetables such as lettuce, spinach, arugula, kale, and/or mixed greens. Keeping the liquid (salad dressing) separate from your leafy vegetables in the jar preserves your healthy salad for three to four days and up to seven days if it is vacuum-sealed.

> **Hint**: Before you close the jar with the lid, place a folded paper towel on top of the salad. Make sure to leave enough room in the jar. The paper towel will absorb excess moisture and keep the leafy vegetables from wilting. Screw the lid on tightly and store in your refrigerator. All the jar needs is a quick shake and you are ready to enjoy!

CRUNCHY BASIL SALAD

Bottom layer:

- 3 tablespoons olive oil
- 3 teaspoons apple cider vinegar
- 2 teaspoons honey
- 2 teaspoons chopped fresh basil
- ½ clove garlic

Combine all ingredients in a small bowl and whisk together then pour into a mason jar.

Middle Layer:

- Cherry Tomatoes
- Orange Bell Peppers
- Red Bell Peppers
- Cucumber
- Shredded Carrots
- Avocado
- Pine Nuts
- Sliced Steak

Top Layer:

- Baby Spinach

Instructions: Add all three layers to the jar in order, starting with the homemade salad dressing at the bottom. Shake and enjoy.

KOREAN SESAME SALAD

Bottom layer:

- 1 tablespoon soy sauce
- 1 teaspoon grated ginger
- 1 tablespoon water
- 1 teaspoon of honey
- 1 tablespoon distilled white vinegar
- 2 teaspoons sesame oil
- 1 teaspoon red pepper flakes

Combine all ingredients in a small bowl and whisk together then pour into a mason jar.

Middle Layer:

- Baby Carrots
- Onion
- Cucumber
- Sugar Snap Peas
- Orange Bell Pepper
- Cherry Tomatoes

Top Layer:

- Lettuce
- Red Cabbage

Instructions: Add all three layers to the jar in order, starting with the homemade salad dressing at the bottom. Shake and enjoy.

SIMPLE SICILIAN SALAD

Bottom layer:

- 3 tablespoons extra virgin olive oil
- 2 tablespoons balsamic vinegar
- 1/2 teaspoon dried oregano
- Salt and pepper to taste

Combine all ingredients in a small bowl and whisk together then pour into a mason jar.

Middle Layer:

- Olives
- Tomatoes
- Pepperoni
- Mozzarella

Top Layer:

- Baby Romaine

Instructions: Add all three layers to the jar in order, starting with the homemade salad dressing at the bottom. Shake and enjoy.

CHINESE CHOPPED SALAD

Bottom layer:

- 6 teaspoons red wine vinegar
- 2 tablespoons extra-virgin olive oil
- 1/2 teaspoon hoisin sauce
- 1/2 teaspoon honey
- 1/4 teaspoon minced garlic
- Salt and ground black pepper to taste

Combine all ingredients in a small bowl and whisk together then pour into a mason jar.

Middle Layer:

- Shredded Carrots
- Bean Sprouts
- Green Onions
- Pear
- Cooked Chicken
- Slivered Almonds

Top Layer:

- Kale
- Baby Spinach

Instructions: Add all three layers to the jar in order, starting with the homemade salad dressing at the bottom. Shake and enjoy.

CLASSIC ITALIAN SALAD

Bottom layer:

- 1 tablespoon apple cider vinegar
- 3 tablespoons olive oil
- 1/4 clove garlic, minced
- 1 teaspoon chopped fresh basil
- 1/4 teaspoon dried oregano
- 1/4 teaspoon of honey

Combine all ingredients in a small bowl and whisk together then pour into a mason jar.

Middle Layer:

- Red Bell Pepper
- Cucumber
- Cherry Tomato
- Red Onion
- Mozzarella
- Pepperoni

Top Layer:

- Baby Spinach

Instructions: Add all three layers to the jar in order, starting with the homemade salad dressing at the bottom. Shake and enjoy.

ASIAN GINGER SALAD

Bottom layer

- 1/2 clove garlic
- 1 teaspoon grated fresh ginger root
- 2 tablespoons olive oil
- 2 teaspoon rice vinegar
- 1 tablespoon soy sauce
- 1 teaspoon honey

Combine all ingredients in a small bowl and whisk together then pour into a mason jar.

Middle Layer:

- Bean Sprouts
- Broccoli
- Sugar Snap Peas
- Apple or Pear
- Shredded Carrots
- Diced Walnuts
- Cooked Turkey

Top Layer:

- Baby Romaine

Instructions: Add all three layers to the jar in order, starting with the homemade salad dressing at the bottom. Shake and enjoy.

HONEY BALSAMIC SALAD

Bottom layer:

- 2 teaspoons balsamic vinegar
- 1/4 small onion, chopped
- 1 teaspoon soy sauce
- 3 teaspoons honey
- 1/2 clove garlic, minced
- 3 tablespoons extra-virgin olive oil

Combine all ingredients in a small bowl and whisk together then pour into a mason jar.

Middle Layer:

- Broccoli
- Sugar Snap Peas
- Diced Avocado
- Sliced Steak
- Orange Pepper

Top Layer:

- Spinach
- Red Cabbage

Instructions: Add all three layers to the jar in order, starting with the homemade salad dressing at the bottom. Shake and enjoy.

CHAPTER 27:
MIX AND MATCH MEALS

Mix and match the breakfasts, lunches and dinners in this book, add different snacks and you'll never feel deprived or bored with your 'diet'—it's *Easy Eating* at its best, as calories are controlled but flavor is out of control!

It's up to you; when you eat the *Easy Eating* way, you're the boss and you are going to burn fat. Enjoy whatever foods you like, including bread and pasta but be sure to put those carbohydrates to good use by getting four or five good workouts a week.

TIPS:

- Mix and match simple snacks like 1 cup of raspberries with 1 square of dark chocolate, for just 150 calories. Yum!

- Mix and match busy breakfasts like sliced pear and almond-butter toast for 350 calories. Yum!

- Mix and match lean lunches like an avocado and black-bean wrap for 400 calories. Yum!

- Mix and match delectable dinners like garlic-basil shrimp and zucchini pasta for 450 calories. Yum!

MIX AND MATCH MENU PLANNER
350-CALORIE BREAKFAST CHOICES

Whole-Grain Walnut Waffles with Berries

- 2 frozen low-fat whole-grain waffles
- 1/4 cup blackberries
- 1/4 cup strawberries
- 1 ounce (14 halves) walnuts

Make it: Toast waffles. Top with mashed fresh berries and walnuts.

Easy English Egg Scramble

- 2 eggs
- 1/2 cup fresh spinach
- 1 whole-grain or sprouted grain English muffin, toasted
- 1 cup cut cantaloupe

Make it: Scramble eggs with spinach. Serve on English muffin with cantaloupe on the side.

Sliced Apple & Almond-Butter Toast

- 1 slice whole-or sprouted grain bread
- 1 tablespoon almond butter
- 1 apple, sliced

Make it: Toast whole-grain bread. Spread almond butter on toast and top with fresh apple slices.

Crunchy Cherry Cereal

- 1 cup unsweetened vanilla almond milk
- 1/2 cup old-fashioned oatmeal
- 1/4 cup dried cherries
- sprinkle of crushed walnuts

   Make it: Pour almond milk on raw old-fashioned oats (prepare the night before and keep in the fridge overnight for softer oats or microwave). Mix in dried tart cherries and nuts.

Tomato-Basil Ricotta Toast

- 1 slice whole-or sprouted grain bread
- 1/2 cup low-fat ricotta cheese
- 5 fresh basil leaves
- 4 slices tomato

   Make it: Toast whole-grain bread. Spread with low-fat ricotta cheese and top with fresh basil leaves and tomato slices

Simple & Sweet Smoothie

- 1 cup unsweetened vanilla almond milk
- 1 scoop of vanilla protein powder
- 1 small banana
- 1 tablespoon honey
- 2 tablespoons old-fashioned oatmeal
- 1 tablespoon flaxseeds, ground

   Make it: Blend all ingredients until smooth.

Lemon-Blueberry Breakfast Granola

- 3/4 cup blueberries
- 1 cup plain Greek yogurt
- 1-ounce crunchy granola or protein bar

  Make it: Top blueberries with yogurt and crushed granola bar. Add a drop of lemon juice.

400-CALORIE LUNCH CHOICES

BBQ Burger & Slaw

- 1 fresh or leftover cooked burger patty
- 1 whole-grain hamburger bun or lettuce wrap
- 1 tablespoon of bbq sauce and mustard
- 1 1/2 cups shredded cabbage, broccoli, cauliflower and carrot mix
- 1 tablespoon apple-cider vinegar
- 2 teaspoons olive oil

  Make it: Microwave burger until warm. Serve on bun with condiments. Combine vegetable mix with vinegar and oil.

Tasty Tuna, Grape & Walnut Salad

- 2 cups of mixed greens salad
- 3 ounces white chunk albacore tuna
- 3 tablespoons chopped walnuts
- 3/4 cup red grapes, cut in half
- 2 tablespoons vinaigrette dressing

Make it: Top greens with tuna, walnuts, and grapes. Drizzle with vinaigrette.

Takeout Treat! *From Your Favorite Fast Food Restaurant*

- Choose the smallest regular burger, sandwich, sub or wrap they have, pair with a small side salad with low-fat balsamic vinaigrette.
- Water or diet soda to drink.

Turkey, Pear & Swiss Sandwich

- 1 teaspoon Dijon mustard
- 2 slices whole-grain bread
- 5 thin slices natural deli turkey
- 1 medium pear, sliced
- 1 slice low-fat Swiss cheese

Make it: Spread mustard on bread. Top with turkey, fresh pear slices, and cheese.

Avocado & Black-Bean Wrap

- 1 whole wheat tortilla
- 1/4 cup canned black beans, rinsed and drained
- 1/4 avocado, chopped
- 2 tablespoons bottled salsa
- 1 cup bagged romaine lettuce

Make it: Wrap black beans, avocado, salsa, and lettuce in tortilla.

Balsamic Chicken Salad Pita

- 1 cup precooked and diced chicken breast
- 2 tablespoons balsamic vinegar
- 1/4 cup chopped scallions
- 1 large stalk celery, chopped
- 1 whole wheat pita
- 1 cup bagged mixed salad greens

Make it: Mix together chicken, vinegar, scallions, and celery. Fill pita with chicken mixture and salad greens.

Personal Pizza

- 1 whole-grain or sprouted grain English muffin, toasted
- 2 tablespoons of marinara sauce
- 3 tablespoons of mozzarella cheese
- 1/4 cup chopped peppers and mushrooms

Make it: spread on sauce, top with cheese and veggies. Broil or warm in microwave

450-CALORIE DINNER CHOICES

Takeout! From Your Favorite Restaurant

- **Grilled Chicken or Cobb Salad** with balsamic vinaigrette dressing.
- Lemon ice water or diet soda to drink.

Garlic-Basil Shrimp & Zucchini Pasta

- 1 cup of sprialized zucchini noodles
- 3 ounces frozen precooked and shelled shrimp, thawed
- 2 tablespoons chopped fresh basil
- 2 garlic cloves, minced
- 1 tablespoon olive oil

Make it: Sauté noodles with remaining ingredients.

Spicy Peanut Chicken Wraps

- 2/3 cup precooked chicken breast
- 1/4 cup chopped scallions
- 2 tablespoons peanuts
- 1 tablespoon hot sauce
- 1 cup shredded cabbage, broccoli, cauliflower and carrot mix
- 2 whole wheat tortillas

Make it: In skillet sprayed with cooking spray, saute chicken, scallions, peanuts, hot sauce, and shredded vegetables for 8 minutes. Wrap in tortillas. Eat one, save one for next day meal.

Takeout! Sushi

- Your favourite Sushi roll (6 pieces)

Three-Pepper Fast Fajitas

- 1/3 cup each sliced red, green and yellow bell peppers
- 1/2 small onion, sliced
- 1 tablespoon olive oil
- 1/2 cup canned refried beans
- 2 whole wheat tortillas
- 1/4 cup cilantro, chopped

Make it: Saute peppers and onion in olive oil for 8 minutes, or until tender. Warm refried beans; spread on tortillas. Top with sauteed vegetables and cilantro. Eat one, save one for next day meal.

Artichoke & Tomato Panzanella Salad

- 1 slices whole-grain bread
- 1/2 cup chopped canned artichokes, rinsed and drained
- 1/2 cup chopped fresh tomato
- 1/4 cup canned white beans, rinsed and drained
- 2 tablespoons low-fat Italian vinaigrette dressing

Make it: Toast bread and cut into small squares. Add artichokes, tomatoes, white beans, toasted bread squares, and Italian vinaigrette and combine.

Hoisin Grilled Fish & Vegetables

- 4 ounces fish, such as salmon, cod or tilapia fillets
- 1 tablespoon hoisin sauce (Chinese barbecue sauce found in the Asian section of grocery stores)
- 1/2 cup chopped yellow squash
- 1/2 cup pea pods
- 1/2 cup chopped carrots
- 2/3 cup cooked brown rice

Make it: Spray a sheet of tin foil with cooking spray and place fish, hoisin sauce, yellow squash, pea pods, and carrots on it. Fold and seal. Cook packet on grill for 10 to 12 minutes (vegetables should be tender and fish should flake easily with a fork). Serve over brown rice.

150-CALORIE SNACK CHOICES

Eating between meals can be fine to hold off hunger as long as you control your portions and it's been proven to make you eat less during your main meals. Choose one or two of these snack options—each is approximately 150 calories.

- 1/2 ounce raisins and 2 tablespoons peanuts
- 1 small serving pack of 2% Greek yogurt
- 12 almonds and a small apple
- 1 cup raspberries with 1 square of 70-90% dark chocolate
- 1 scoop of protein powder shaken in water
- 1 ounce chocolate-covered almonds
- 6 whole grain or gluten free crackers topped with cheddar cheese
- 100-calorie mini bag popcorn
- 1 ounce string cheese and 10 pistachios
- 1/4 cup hummus and 1/2 cup baby carrots
- Root beer float! (1/4 cup vanilla frozen yogurt, 12 ounces diet root beer)

Made in the USA
Lexington, KY
21 November 2018